1965

DOUBLE
YOUR ENERGY
AND LIVE
WITHOUT FATIGUE

Other Books by Margery Wilson

CHARM

YOUR PERSONALITY AND GOD

MAKE UP YOUR MIND

THE WOMAN YOU WANT TO BE

THE NEW ETIQUETTE

HOW TO LIVE BEYOND YOUR MEANS

BE YOURSELF

I FOUND MY WAY

DOUBLE YOUR ENERGY AND LIVE WITHOUT FATIGUE

by

Margery Wilson

Prentice-Hall, Inc.
Englewood Cliffs, N.J.

Library of Congress Catalog Number: 61-14360

First printing......September, 1961
Second printing....November, 1961
Third printing...... February, 1962
Fourth printing ....May, 1962
Fifth printing ....July, 1962
Sixth printing........January, 1963

Printed in the United States of America

21880-T

THIS BOOK IS DEDICATED TO MY DAUGHTER ELIZABETH WHOSE GROW-
ING-UP TAUGHT ME MUCH OF HUMAN ENDURANCE AND REACTION.

Contents

DOUBLE
YOUR ENERGY
AND LIVE
WITHOUT FATIGUE

1

⚭ ⚭

READ THIS FIRST

Would you like to have twice the energy you now have? Wouldn't it be fine to have the extra drive to do all the things you would like to do? Does that idea appeal to you? Wouldn't you like to have twice the endurance you have today? Wouldn't you like to be able to say, "I am stronger now than I was ten years ago. I do not know what real exhaustion is like! Yes, I do get sleepy at times and I enjoy my sleep, but I cannot say that my body is ever completely emptied of energy, or that my mind is truly tired."

Then, follow me through this book. Let me share with you my experiences with energy versus fatigue. I know what it is to be so tired that the very marrow of my bones seems to throb faintly with weakness. There is no angle of weariness that I cannot understand. That is why I would like to give every tired person in the world the help for this problem that I gained for myself.

You do not have to be tired. You can gain the upper hand over this most vicious enemy of modern society, fatigue. At a tender age, it became apparent to me that one must pull away from weakness or be forever trapped by it. The truth is that I was simply fed up with it. The idea of being "delicate" had become fastened upon me. Being very thin and subject to colds, my mother's acute concern had put me, bit by bit, with those "people apart" who mustn't overdo and must take the most boring care of themselves. None of this design-for-dwindling fitted into that dream-pattern of a charming and elegant female that fills the head of every girl-child. Thoroughly out of patience

1

with all this pampering hampering, I decided (due to my father's encouraging statements that one could become whatever one wished to be) that I was going to be strong, healthy and never, *never* be without energy. How well I succeeded is best known to my family, my friends and my employees who try to keep up with me. This book invites you to free yourself from your most formidable enemy—tiredness.

Fatigue is the popular, the fashionable, the universal disease! People who meet on the street never fail to tell each other how tired they are. It has come to be the expected response to "How are you?" The answer is a surprising "I'm simply dead!" Two men will explain to each other, quite seriously, their exact state of tiredness. And having exchanged this mouldy bit of news, they seem to think that they have had a proper conversation, and will say "good-bye" with the warmest manner.

There is a tacit understanding that the admission of fatigue was a confidence, but both of them will forget that bit of nonsense as soon as they meet someone else to whom they can tell, confidentially, how tired they are. And so it goes. Men should recall the briefing given by the State Department to all ambassadors, ministers and their aides. "Never say that you are tired. You represent your country as you go about abroad. Your country must not be pictured as exhausted!"

Listen also to women. Two women will meet and say exactly what the men have said, but it is even less becoming to them. Women are supposed to supply the freshness, the encouragement, that nourishes life. To them I will say, "Be careful of your words. If you keep saying you're dead, sooner or later somebody is going to believe you and say behind your back, 'Well, I guess the old girl is done for!' "

Mrs. Eleanor Roosevelt has often said that almost the first thing she learned about public life was that she must never say she was tired. One wonders if that discipline was not the forerunner of the gathering of her prodigious energy that is still the marvel of her associates. Her program, today, would stagger many a younger person.

How do you advertise yourself? In a society where advertising proves our belief in the repeated suggestion, it is astonishing that both men and women will underrate themselves by stating many times a day that they are worn out and failing fast! Almost everyone does it.

What of the effect on yourself? The suggestion of being spent is deadly since it falls on a hearer's ears, but what about the force of this suggestion in the subconscious mind of the speaker? We will examine this thought in detail later in the book. All of which brings us again to the important fact—

Almost all the people with extraordinary energy, have, somewhere along the line, decided to have it. One thing is certain, if one does not decide to have it, energy seems to tip-toe away as did the old Persian gods—"who depart on feet of wool, we do not hear them go." Apparently, energy must be invited, demanded, articulated, asserted deep within oneself. Many people have arrived at this demand for various reasons and at different times in their lives. Some people seem "naturally" attuned to energy, others, most of us, must be deliberate about it. But the laws of energy are quite the same, whether they are approached with a plan in mind or just "natural" exuberance. Like all laws, they respond to anyone, saint or sinner, who meets their requirements, much as does electricity.

You can use the laws of energy. It matters not, at the beginning, whether you are a tired businessman who drives his brain for hours on end every day and night, or a weak little woman who simply can't find the strength to keep ahead of her housework, a person with a record of depleting illnesses, or a youngster whose studies and work are an overloading challenge to his limited energies. There is more energy for *you.* You will find that as it flows into you, the extra blessings of life will miraculously accompany or follow it.

Extra energy is like a genie who grants your wishes. It is fatigue that causes people to think they cannot go ahead with the effort to train themselves along the lines of their fine talents. *Extra* energy would make that road of preparation seem only a happy, exciting challenge. Each day's reward of extra skill in return for the effort put into a dream would put you ahead on the ever more smooth path to your goal.

Fatigue is the real "boss" in many a life. It makes a man think he can't have an avocation. When he comes home, he's dead-tired. He is convinced that he must "rest" when he isn't working at his major job. He has no enthusiasm for his children's lives, nor can he take any part in them. Insidiously, fatigue takes over the rule of his entire life. The romance he once had with his wife, seeing his friends, fun, extra learning, *everything* must be sacrificed on the altar of his fatigue. He lives a life of diminshing returns.

Extra energy provides a life of accruing values. There is extra fun, extra work, extra recognition, extra money, extra generosity, all adding up to a fuller life. Fulfillment, for a youngster or an oldster, often hangs on one word—energy!

A reserve of strength gives one more patience. Thus, more courtesy makes one seem more charming. (The sharp retort is often just a bark from that old dog, fatigue.) One can make the small extra effort that may open up new fields of profit. The extra telephone call may help a friend or gain one. By listening an extra moment to someone's story, one gives and gets new depths of understanding. Writing an extra note for business or pleasure can be a magic touch that extends a man's influence and multiplies his accomplishment and happiness.

But, if he is already exhausted (or thinks he is) he will push it all away from him, sag in the middle, go home to "grump" at the family, or disappear into a silence that is like a pall. Most people in this state have nothing organically wrong with them. They want desperately the vigor that makes life more fascinating. Many doctors tell them the truth, that—

Only they can correct the causes of their tiredness. But how can the average man acquire the extra strength to defy the fatigue that keeps him from greater success in living? Science, experiment and growing knowledge point to the fact that he can find it right within himself. But he must reinterpret, reallocate, entirely redefine his energies until he understands and commands them. He will master his body, and not let it master him!

Growing knowledge comes from many sources. There is considerable help coming from the field of medical research.

Dr. Peter Krohn of England, a Nobel Prize winner, has done a great deal of work in the field of geriatrics (the study of why the human being grows tired, old and dies so soon). There are many other distinguished men and teams of men working for enlightenment on the problem.

Most of our foundations, our universities and many individual scientists are devoting much time and millions of dollars to the study of the epidemic disease of fatigue. The general assumption is that we need not bow under its rule—that we can conquer it, but also, that each man must assume responsibility for himself. About twenty of our research groups compared their findings several years ago and all agreed that the best definition of fatigue they could agree, upon, so far, is—

"AN UNWILLINGNESS TO CONTINUE LONGER UNDER
THE EXISTING CIRCUMSTANCES"

Exhaustion, they say, is difficult to pin down. A new factor brought into most experiments will show that there is at least one more (and perhaps many) bursts of energy in a seemingly spent muscle, mind, or man.

The secret lies in a combination of factors. No single approach to the goal of increased energy can be said to be conclusive. There are a number of paths, all within the reach of anyone who really wants to conquer fatigue. And I have tried most of them! Physical culture, rest, drugs, diet, Yoga, massage, color therapy, music therapy, and many others! I found some merit in each of them. I also found contradictions.

PANACEAS AND CONTRADICTIONS

In the field of diet, there were those who said that only milk was the perfect way to health. Others said that milk was virtually poison. I drank gallons of milk and ignored it by turns. There were those who said that meat was not fit for the human body, and others who claimed that only meat supplied the body's voracious appetite for protein. I was a vegetarian and a meat-eater by turns.

At one point, somebody whispered to me that the ailing

popes and kings had been kept alive by a special diet of embryos, theoretically filled with the promises of developing life. Obediently, I ate hundreds of eggs, only to hear later that eggs would surely kill anyone who ate a vast quantity of them.

Then, my mother heard that the Scottish women were lovely looking and rosy with health, the men very strong, because they ate great quantities of oatmeal. Following this pronouncement, we lived in a sea of oatmeal preparations for years! Are there now any among us who do not know of the cult of juices, vegetable and fruit juices, that contain the elixir of life? And now we are in the honey and vinegar age.

As an ardent guinea-pig, I have tried on myself many systems, notions and cults. I found them all good. Perhaps I was saved from disaster by changing to something else before the ill effects of any particular excess could harm me. If a sly note of levity has crept in here, let me say very seriously, that there seems to be no doubt of the value of proper food. A great deal is known about it. Besides, it is one of the delights of life. The pleasure it gives is one of its benefits. In fact, most of the things you will be asked to do in order to multiply your energies, are extremely pleasant, once you get the hang of them.

Fatigue is not imaginary. It is a very real condition, even when its causes are in the mind. We should understand its reality very clearly. Just gritting your teeth and making an extra effort when you think you are tired, is sometimes worse than nothing. For so long as you are in the grip of the whole fabric of fatigue, you can harm yourself by adding to your exhaustion.

Be gentle with yourself. If you are tired, it is because of a complication of reasons. We must unravel them before your energies are freed. We are going to take this whole subject apart and show you, bit by bit, how the structure of your fatigue was built, and how you can set about replacing it with a fine acquisition of energy.

Then you will be searching out ways to spend your surging "electrical" charge. Your creative urges will rise again in your mind and lure you on to new goals full of *life*. That extra appointment, that understanding smile, that dance with your hostess (or host), that speech you were asked to give, that creative money-saving or money-making work at home, all those and hundreds of other things can be yours.

And what about that big dream of being someone important to the world? You will have energy for that, too. The more you examine the subject of energy, the more clearly you will see that it is ever-present. It is we who cut ourselves off from it. It is we who can find it again. *I Did! And If I Did—You Can!*

Let me begin by stating my premise and some of its supporting ideas.

A HUMAN BEING HAS POWERS BEYOND THOSE OF THE VEGETABLE AND THE ANIMAL

Consider the concept that all forms of life are designed in separate, unique patterns. Under normal conditions, each has the energy to fulfill its design and become the finished expression of its seed's potential.

Vegetable life obviously moves to its fruition, and then it withers. But man is not a vegetable. In animal life, we see the inherent pattern of each individual in any given species develop according to its design, gradually empty itself of energy, and die.

Man is generally classed as a superior animal. He has the capacity to adjust himself to his environment, and even to change his environment somewhat—outside and beyond the animal pattern.

How far, and in what ways he may leave it behind in his growing awareness, lie in the hands of each individual man.

It would be foolish to say that he is not bound by the physical laws of his animal existence, but it is not foolish to say that this is not all he may become.

He can transcend the laws of his animal life by first obeying them (at least, not flouting them) and thus, become master of them. A good analogy lies in the field of electricity. By first obeying its laws, we become master of it, and use it as we will—for cold, heat, power, light, or whatever.

The power man possesses, which is beyond his animal cycle

of presently known experience, has been called by many names, more popularly mind, or soul. Whatever it is, he has it! Thus, man need not bow under the yoke of his so-called physical limitations. He stands facing infinity and he has a mind to probe it.

With this much granted, we have a basis for drawing on (or, if you prefer, releasing) extra power. Naturally, it takes a little time to learn how to do so. Meanwhile, there is much we can do right where we are, to help ourselves win that daily battle with fatigue. There is quite a span between man's possible strength and his present performance, but one need not wait to know and understand the entire matter before he can gain some relief and benefit.

YOUR HISTORY HOLDS THE REASONS FOR YOUR PRESENT

Millions of years are required to build an awareness in an animal, or any form of life. Instinct is said (though the subject is moot) to be simply the result of a long, long background of accumulated experience.

The memory of repeated results down through time (buried in the interaction of glands, nerves and marrow) finally builds an acceptance of a pattern into the unconscious mental and physical reflexes of a creature. These acceptances become the "way he will function" at his present point in evolution.

We, as we stand today, are the result of millions (perhaps more) of years of certain patterns of being and behavior. We progress so very slowly, largely because we do so little thinking, choosing or initiating. We develop more animal "cunning" than independent intelligence because we usually think only expediently on immediate problems. The tendency to expediency is inherent, because man, for eons of time, was a nomad seeking food and always and only an immediate advantage. Expediency retarded and still retards man's larger advances. He still acts upon the thing he confronts at any given moment without much analysis or projection. In his immature reactions he grabs, as an infant does, at whatever he likes, regardless of to whom it belongs. This inherited tendency obscures the fact that he has the power to *create* something better for himself. In many areas he still reacts expediently, especially in immaturely accepting his status instead of using his mind to correct it.

Thus, a habit or trait, with roots millions of years old, becomes a compulsion in time. Much that man thinks about his world and himself is based on false or outmoded sense testimony, but he seldom has the mental energy to throw off its thralldom and to find the facts that would free him from his animal limits. It is now necessary for him to emerge from that imprisoning past. Each man must make his own break with the well-established mass-hypnosis of personal weakness—fatigue.

By the gathered suggestion of long-repeated results, man has come to rationalize fatigue and to accept it. But it is actually no more necessary to accept than for him to carry a club and live in a cave. It belongs to the past when he may have been more helpless than he is today.

It is now important for him to conquer the inherent tendency to fatigue, in order that he may survive in the new world he is discovering.

Man is finding amazing powers in his outer world. He must balance them with the remarkable powers he can find within himself. He must decide which habits he has unprofitably brought along (and actually defended) and be brave enough to discard the useless ones. Thus, we will progress one more notch from the animal state.

FATIGUE IS LARGELY A BAD HABIT, FOSTERED FOR COMPLICATED REASONS. YOU, MY READER, ARE CLEVER ENOUGH TO DISCARD IT.

2

YOUR FATIGUE HABITS

AREN'T YOU TIRED OF BEING TIRED?

What are your fatigue habits? There are definite patterns of reaction that most of us have set up for ourselves, and they are quite dependable! Each person has his own projected plan of how he will get through a day. He has a fairly good idea of just how he will feel as the day progresses. He should, he thinks. He has been going through his routine for a long time.

Suppose we begin with your waking moment, any morning, and analyze your average day. You are likely to belong to one of three types of people, or some combination of them.

TYPE 1.

You awake refreshed, full of energy, joy and go quickly to dress. A song bubbles to your lips. You sometimes sing in the shower. Whatever you think the day holds, stimulates your energies in anticipation. You can hardly wait to get out to see what wonders this day may offer.

(This fortunate individual doesn't even think of fatigue. He doesn't, therefore, plan ahead to be tired at, say, eleven o'clock.)

TYPE 2.

You find it difficult to awake, and sometimes feel as though you had been beaten all night with a stick. After groaning and creaking for a few minutes, you finally loosen up enough to get up.

10

(This person may have a physical as well as an emotional cause for his state of depletion. He would do well to find the real reason for it.)

TYPE 3.

You awake slowly and lie dreading the efforts of the day. You sigh, remembering the dull routine of past days. You wonder why your life is so uninteresting. The small ache in your heart is remembered hurt. You lie there and gather into your mind the several slights and neglects you suffer from those nearest you. Why doesn't someone offer you love, solace, companionship? You hover between despair and hope, then you finally hurry into your clothes. You dress your body, but not your mind, or your expression. You go out into the world with an empty, sad face; you sit in your car, or on a bus, and mull over your low estate. Many other people are doing the same thing, but you scarcely notice them.

(This individual's name is legion. His routine is that of the millions of people who are, or think they are tired. These people look at their clocks every morning, think over their jobs or errands for the day and say to themselves, "I know I shall be dead tired by one o'clock. I shall be needing some coffee to prop me up. I'd better wear some loose, old shoes." Note that these tired ones have already put old shoes and the little brown coffee bean in the place of vigor and well-being. Any old thing can be enthroned when one abdicates as ruler of his own body and life!)

At what hour do you expect to be tired? This is an honest question and deserves an honest answer. Look at yourself in the mirror any morning and ask yourself how long you REALLY EXPECT to feel adequate to whatever you will be doing. Are you a ten o'clock, eleven o'clock or after-lunch failure? Or—

Can you anticipate being full of vigor at five in the afternoon? Will you still be charged with energy enough to go home to some work or sport until dinner, after which you expect to study or play games, or dance, or go visiting until a proper bedtime?

Most of humanity *expects* to be defeated by fatigue at some special hour during the day, and from then on to play at dodging duty, avoiding life, short-changing the job, or whatever. At what hour do *you* expect to be defeated, and yield the honors to fatigue?

MAKE YOUR OWN ENERGY CHART

A.M. 6-7-8-9-10-11-Noon- 1-2-3-4-5-6-7-8-9-10-11- Midnight

On the next two pages you will find an example of one. Chart your own energy.

Now study your chart. Is it as you would like it to be? What is responsible for its low points? Is there a cause, a real cause, or is it just a bad habit? Are you following someone else's example? What simple means could you employ to keep your energy line high? Could you eliminate these low points entirely? Do you believe that you can raise them, quickly— slowly—?

Some real soul-searching is necessary to arrive at the truth. You need not take me, or anyone else, into your confidence. In fact, I advise against sweeping admissions to anyone except yourself, but it is important for you not to deceive yourself. I ask you the following suggestions, not to "needle" you, but to help you to see yourself and your problems as clearly as possible. You must make some decisions before you can make plans.

1. DECIDE whether your low points are caused by physical or emotional drains. If your needs are beyond your knowledge, get professional help, in either area.
2. DECIDE whether habit has you in a vise. Habit is an illusion of necessity. Good habits, as well as bad ones, can be formed in two or three weeks. Cultivate the habit of thinking of energy, not of fatigue.
3. DECIDE whether you really want to call attention to the great effort you put into life. Being tired is one way to do so. No grown person should hobble himself with this bit of childishness, but millions of us take this method of dramatizing ourselves. What a costly bit of by-play!

Check the flow of your energy with this
ENERGY METER

See instructions on other side

MONDAY { High / Med. / Low }

A.M.							P.M.												
6	7	8	9	10	11	12	1	2	3	4	5	6	7	8	9	10	11	12

TUESDAY { High / Med. / Low }

A.M.							P.M.												
6	7	8	9	10	11	12	1	2	3	4	5	6	7	8	9	10	11	12

WEDNESDAY { High / Med. / Low }

A.M.							P.M.												
6	7	8	9	10	11	12	1	2	3	4	5	6	7	8	9	10	11	12

THURSDAY { High / Med. / Low }

A.M.							P.M.												
6	7	8	9	10	11	12	1	2	3	4	5	6	7	8	9	10	11	12

FRIDAY { High / Med. / Low }

A.M.							P.M.												
6	7	8	9	10	11	12	1	2	3	4	5	6	7	8	9	10	11	12

SATURDAY { High / Med. / Low }

A.M.							P.M.												
6	7	8	9	10	11	12	1	2	3	4	5	6	7	8	9	10	11	12

SUNDAY { High / Med. / Low }

A.M.							P.M.												
6	7	8	9	10	11	12	1	2	3	4	5	6	7	8	9	10	11	12

Easy Instructions for Using Your
ENERGY METER

In order to fight fatigue you must know its weakest point. The most accurate way to find this point is to give yourself a test on the ENERGY METER for a 7-day period. It's easy to keep your record as described below:

1. Look at the example at the bottom of the page. When you complete your testing, the chart will look something like this.
2. Keep your ENERGY METER (or a copy of it) in a convenient place and within easy reach, so that you can record your degree of energy at ·regular intervals.
3. Now, begin to clock your energy levels by placing a dot in the square marked high, medium or low. Use only one dot for the hour you are recording.
4. After you have completed your tabulation for one day, connect all the dots with one line. After a few days you will notice the fluctuation of the line, whether it dips or rises at specific hours during the day.

When you have completed the 7-day ENERGY METER test, compare the results and then ask yourself these questions:

- How can I change my fatigue-hour, or even eliminate it entirely? — Chapter 2 of *Double Your Energy and Live Without Fatigue tells you how.*
- Are my mental energies drained by emotional fatigue from thinking about the past?—See Chapter 7
- Can knowing my energy levels help me to make new friends and keep old ones? —Chapter 13 reveals the startling facts.
- Is it possible for me to give energy to other people? —Read Chapter 14

Example: { High Med. Low }

4. DECIDE whether you secretly *like* to be the object of sympathetic understanding and concern. One can easily bog down in it.

5. DECIDE to win inner comfort and outer admiration for your energetic performance. You need nobody's sympathy or lack-luster recognition. Everybody who knows you knows the fine effort you are making, or have made. He who runs may read. Why try so hard, so immaturely—and at such a cost—to establish an obvious fact?

6. DECIDE not to "sell your birthright for a mess of pottage," *i.e.* the highly questionable pleasures that come with fatigue. Your natural position as a strong, mature person has much more to give you!

Now you see how extremely important is complete honesty with yourself. Defending your status, your practices, putting the blame on something or somebody else, excusing yourself, explaining away your power "to do anything about it" simply delay any correction.

Take command of yourself and demand of your body a more satisfactory performance every day. Let me draw your attention to the fact that you, and you alone, can direct the processes of your body. You did not originate it, any more than you built the car you drive, but if you don't drive both machines well, you will wind up with a couple of wrecks. You are the driver. You are at the controls. There is no way that anyone else can get into your organism in its interaction.

If you are not commanding your citadel, it is without a general. Certain "natural" patterns will fulfill themselves in you and your life, but unless *you* supply the conscious demand into which you can draw the energy of natural force, it simply completes it cycle, its pattern, as a vegetable does!

You have chosen whatever you have. If you do not command your body you have chosen a *laissez-faire* attitude in which any old thing can happen. If you do demand of yourself a better performance, according to established laws, you know the deep satisfaction of their obedience to your directive.

Now, let us return to your day, and the way you feel at some given hour. Whatever you feel, it is largely, as we have stated, your own choice. Whether or not you admit it, *you* have established a pattern for your body to follow. Having no volition of its own, it follows this directed pattern. If you tell it to be tired at eleven o'clock, at three or five o'clock, it will oblige you, having no alternative.

Again—there is nobody in there with you to influence your decision to be tired. Within you, there is the full force of mind's shaping power. Life and mind are within you, and they are far better for you than "somebody." The force of life is, in a sense, like a powerful presence in which we live and move and have our being. It is there, available, waiting, ready to fulfill your mental pattern.

The life-force within you does not compel you to choose one design or another. It flows into and takes the form you hold up for it, much as gelatin takes the shape of the mold into which it is poured. (Pardon the homely illustration.) What is your mental-pattern, your mold of your body? What are you telling it to become? Are you accepting the world-thought of fatigue, or are you acting as an individual creator (with "dominion" over your world yourself)?

Make this experiment. Look at a clock tomorrow morning and mentally say to yourself, "I shall assert my God-given right to determine my own condition this day. I shall not be tired at three, four or five o'clock. Since when did a clock (a bit of machinery invented by the mind of man) gain ascendancy over me? That clock is there for the order of my life as a convenience, not as a whip, or a master. I am master of that clock. If I find pleasure in my day's work, I shall gain energy from it!

"I shall have more strength at five o'clock this afternoon than I had at ten this morning. Why not? Why should I bow under the mistaken thought of men, who, in thousands of years, have not thought through to the truth of energy. For thousands of years, they thought the earth was flat! Now they all think their energies are flat. But, I do not think so, and I refuse to follow, like a sheep, this untruth about my being!"

If I could hear you say that, I would be a very happy person, and would silently say to you "Bravo!" For when you find the truth about one thing, it is likely that you will find it in other areas, too.

But do not make rules for others. Do not judge other people by your own new-found release. Remember how much tenacity there is in a habit-thought that is thousands, perhaps millions, of years old. Do not make unfair, unjust demands on others, who are enmeshed in the old, intricate and tyrannical forms of fatigue.

Be gentle with those who believe in fatigue. Making fun of them will get you nothing but their undying hate. They will take every means to find you wrong. And being human yourself, they will probably find your weak point, use it to prick you, and nothing will be gained.

NEVER TAKE A "SUPERIOR" ATTITUDE BECAUSE YOU HAVE A NEW VIEW OF YOUR ENERGIES

If you really want to help others, just keep pointing to their superb vitality when they are pleased. They will work, or play, for hours, untired, if there is constructive pleasure in whatever they are doing. It is up to you to make their efforts a pleasant experience.

I feel fortunate. The extra energy I have discovered in my own body and mind makes me feel, not superior, but very, very fortunate—as though I had found oil in my front yard, and gold in my backyard. To know and to say that it is available to everybody will keep your thinking on a polite and even keel. In any case, people will be far more impressed by what you do than by what you say.

Begin by putting your fatigue-hour ahead by one hour today. If you are customarily tired at eleven o'clock in the morning, *decide* not to be tired until noon. You will have the surprise of your life finding your body obeying the demands you put upon it.

You can push your fatigue-hour ahead one or two hours a week. In two months time you can be free of daytime tiredness. Just keep on pushing. In two more months you can push even the *idea* of fatigue off your agenda entirely. You will get sleepy at a good bedtime, but your body will never be exhausted, never feel completely spent. You will forget to say, "I'm tired." You will not *be* tired.

WARNING!

Do not overexert yourself in any way, now, or you may come to harm. Go very slowly. Do not suddenly decide to run a mile, stay up all night, or lift 200 pounds, in the fatuous belief that you now have control of boundless energy. The ability to do any or all of these things is a matter of *changing* a number of habits, thoughts, approaches and attitudes, really changing even your automatic reactions, not merely making a few grudging concessions, or conversational points. Build your new concepts slowly, safely, and well.

A MATTER OF CONCEPT

The great truth about the body, that is coming to be recognized, is that like the rest of the material world, it operates upon energy released by *ideas*. This energy takes the form of the mental patterns that released it. In turn, these patterns respond to motivating ideas.

How long and how bitterly so-called "material scientists" have fought this conclusion is known to all students. But, one by one, most of its opponents have been won over to the facts which seem unavoidable, *i.e.* the response of nature's powers and processes to the directing mind of man. Psychosomatic medicine is a direct outgrowth of the extending acceptance of these truths. (One even wonders if they aren't overdoing it!)

The battle between the "mechanistic theory" and the "volitional premise" is still on. I do not see that one refutes the other! By *volition* we set into operation certain *mechanistic* processes. Both are here for the use of man. Why not keep both benefits! No one has yet found the outer periphery of either law. Einstein probably could have found a distant point where they merge!

But we are here to benefit, not to argue. One thing is certain —if in too much doubt, fear, or despair, we give over what authority we have found in man's mind to the tyranny of matter, we shall lose all the gains given us by sages and philosophers, down through time. They have seen clearly many truths we regard today as "new."

Here and there a man has called out his wisdom, and all too often, he has been cut down in derision and contempt. Mankind does not change or improve very willingly, it seems. How long, how often must we hear a truth, before we begin to open a crack in our minds for it?

I am not even asking you to consider the proved findings of earnest researchers in ESP (extra-sensory perception). But you may as well brace yourself for a swift unfolding of many of man's higher powers. And one day these "small" matters which we now bridle will be mere details in a past struggle upward to real personal power.

For our purposes—begin to use your power of choice. Choose a brighter picture of and for yourself. Choose the role you will play for the rest of your life, as though you were an actor. Shakespeare wisely said, "All the world's a stage." You are no less an actor just because you have become used to your role. Not only have you chosen your role, your character, but you judge your acts against that concept. You choose your environment to accommodate the character you have selected as yours. The process is so slow that you think it was not volitional. So gradually did you choose the bits and pieces of yourself and your life that you have convinced yourself you are "that way just naturally."

Nevertheless, give some time every day to visualizing yourself as straight, vigorous, supple, graceful, gracious. See yourself strong, gallant and commanding. (Without the counterpart of Walter Mitty in us, we might easily sink back to the jungle.)

Learn your lines. The fine character you choose to play would speak in a certain way that harmonizes with his ideals. What sort of ideas would this fine person you are creating wish to express in words? They would not be incorrect, inappropriate or weak in any way. About 500 B.C. the great Chinese philosopher Confucius said, "Without knowing the force of words, it is impossible to know man."

Choose the fine, truly kindly, rich, sympathetic, encouraging, vigorous words that go with your new "part." This person would spend no time talking about sickness, weakness, failure, disaster or any kind of evil, if he could help it. (If anybody thinks this mode of procedure is "just too sweet for words," let him try it. He will discover that it takes all his strength, discipline, courage and self-control to "make it.")

Choose your words carefully, fastidiously. Eliminate destructive words. Throw them out one at a time. Purify your speech as you would purify the water you drink. Get the deadly germs of all that is dispiriting and fatiguing out of it!

Dress the part you have chosen to play. Costuming is a very important part of any production—and you are producing an energetic, strong, healthy, successful person. Simplicity and quality will be your keynote, as a background for the "go and glow" of yourself. Don't have "company" clothes; do not wear any old thing when you are alone. Remember you are making an impression, a pattern on the becoming, becoming, always becoming sensitive plate of creation. If you give it a picture of "any old thing" that is exactly what you will get back.

Its reflections are as exact (in time) as a mirror's. Do not hold thoughts, attitudes and words of fatigue up to its reflecting, fabricating process. Hold up vigor, fineness, worth and beauty —and only these! Then back them up with faith and tenacity.

For some of us there will be the sound of grinding gears as we try to shift to this new demand. And we will begin to find excuses for ourselves.

Throw out excuses. So you don't have time to go to a gymnasium, or money to take expensive, sunny vacations. No complaints, please! Start at home, or at the office. Buy some iron weights you can lift to train your body to your vigorous pattern.

I know a man who developed wonderful shoulders and a hard stomach with two iron weights in his office. A few minutes with them morning and night *rested* him, he told me. He also had a sun lamp, and ten minutes a day gave him a real tan.

No matter how busy you think you are, you can find a few minutes every day that will give you the muscles, the training, the knowledge and the skills that will help you carry out your new role. Don't take "No" for answer from yourself and you will discover that it will be difficult for the world to say it to you.

Energy to carry out your new demand will reach you from many sources. It will be as though your dynamic idea were a magnet you threw into space and into its trajectory; it will draw what it needs to fulfill itself with enough material, emotional and mental.

True, it will also attract a number of challenges, but they will slink away into the shadows before the continuing sun of your resolve. Tests there will be, but instead of dreading them, you will welcome them. They will be merely hones against which you can sharpen your tools; you will smile at them.

You can say with me, "Draw near cynics, and listen! When you become weary and discouraged, come to me and I will share what I have with you. Don't be ashamed to come. I will not tease you for the attitude you held. I won't even say 'I told you so.' "

3

SOME IMMEDIATE HELP

If you are in earnest about this battle against fatigue, there are three things you will do immediately. Other decisions will come later.

1. Resign from the "cult of the tired."
2. Never, *never* say again "I'm so tired!"
3. Turn your mind to the fact that energy is a *principle,* therefore, is *inexhaustible.*

Mind you, I did not say that *your* energy, as you feel it now, is inexhaustible. I merely ask you to consider that the *principle* of energy is timeless, eternal—as are the principles of love, mathematics, heat and relativity. (Example: One could write the numbers two and four endlessly, as long as one lived. Everybody could do so simultaneously forever, yet the twos and fours could never be exhausted.)

You must feel that you have a source from which you derive your motive power. Otherwise, you will not make claims upon it; just as you would not write checks unless you knew there was an adequate deposit of money to cover them. If you do not conceive of energy as inexhaustible, it can never truly be yours.

But, before we dig deeply into the causes of fatigue, I want to give you some immediate help, suggestions that you can use effectively now. These practices have been gleaned by me in a lifetime search for quick recovery to use in the pressures of my very busy life. They come from swamis and society women, captains of industry, actors on tour, and from my own experiments. Most of them are very simple, but very telling in their effect. They "work"!

Pleasure draws energy. I am writing this book to benefit you, not to draw you into an argument. I simply say try these practices and see for yourself! Let us settle, at once, for the fact that we shall never be perfect in this subject, nor any other, for that matter. Let us also settle for the truth that—

WE ARE SELDOM TIRED BY THE ACTIVITIES THAT REALLY INTEREST US

When we are pleased, we draw energy. When we are displeased we throw it off. Just as a short-circuit will drain electricity from a battery, we become depleted when any type of confusion or inner negation becomes the dominant factor in our lives. These short-circuits within us may be known or unknown, conscious or unconscious. The whys and wherefores come later.

For now, suppose you are extremely tired. A consuming weariness has engulfed your mind and body. Yet, there are duties you must perform, obligations to be met during the rest of the day and evening.

As the French say, your *bête-noir* (black beast) of fatigue creeps to your chair, or to your bedside and seems to live on your energy. There is no time to reorganize your life, to rearrange your emotional set-up. Throw the dog a bone, a practical one! Concede, temporarily, that your body must be refreshed, on purely material lines.

Here are some ways that will bring almost immediate results. (But, remember the real solutions come later.)

1. *The importance of oxygen.* When a patient is sinking, in a hospital, he is given oxygen from a tank for the extra help he needs in his period of shock or depletion. Why wait for the oxygen tank!

Give yourself oxygen by several scientifically perfect, deep breaths. Your entire body needs oxygen. (Vitamin E is said to help hold it in the tissues.) Theoretically, with each heartbeat, the lungs are suffused with blood sent there to be relieved of its poisons, to pick up oxygen, and to take it to the tissues and nerves from your feet to your head.

You can aid this process by cooperating mentally. *Think* of refreshing oxygen going all through you. Draw air deeply into your lungs, fully, slowly. Hold it a moment, and then expel it slowly, forcing out the last. Wait a second or two and then repeat the slow, deep inbreathing. *Think* of the oxygen turning the fatigue gases in your blood stream from blue to red, on contact, as it does in your lungs (or when you cut your finger). New, fresh life is suffusing your body, seeping into every cell. A building and cleansing process is splendidly active within you.

2. *The importance of good posture.* There are three major reasons for straightening up.

A. *The way you look.* Even to yourself. Sagging looks defeated, finished. Uprightness looks vital. It is full of promise.

B. *The way you feel.* Slumping piles your vital organs into a mashed heap in your middle. They cannot function properly. Uprightness gives them room to act and function well.

C. *The way you plan.* Uprightness makes you look as though you had a plan, a project. Indeed, it gives you the steam to project your ideas. Thus, you invite attention and interest.

A quick way to give yourself a straight body, with all its benefits, is to lie down on a hard surface, for two minutes several times a day.

Your entire bone-structure straightens as you lie on your back. Your organs have room to "breathe" and work. A soft bed accepts your fatigue posture and little is accomplished, even in an hour. The slantboards are good, but I cannot get one out and put it away as often as I want the benefit of lying on a good, hard surface.

I lie on the floor several times a day, for two or three minutes. Even in that brief time I can feel my entire body gratefully assuming a vital straightness. The floor seems to push my spinal column into proper position and energy flows into it as though into a magnet. My mind seems cleared and I can think more swiftly. I will not attempt to explain all the salutary reactions of the body. They are so many and so intertwined that I doubt if any one person knows them all. But pressure is definitely removed from the heart, the liver and the digestive tract. Blood circulates gently and easily. Even in two or three minutes, the body gets a fresh start.

Gravity alone, in the course of time, may pull the body down. Age, trouble, confusion, illness and lack of self-respect weigh heavily on the shoulders. The downward sag is the position of emptiness and defeat, an invitation to, as well as an advertisement of, fatigue.

Your body seems to know this automatically, for it acts accordingly. A low chest will make you sad, shy, weak in one or more ways. Your posture, quite naturally, affects your opinion of yourself, almost more than that of the beholder.

3. *The importance of liquids.* In my own experiments with myself and my employees, I learned that a dehydrated muscle is an erratic one. A dehydrated nerve is a jumpy one. An habitually dehydrated body holds not only a residue of left-over poisons, it is also the seat of emotional conflicts. Not having moisture enough seems to contribute to a feeling of inferiority. It ties in with the idea of not having enough of something, or so it appears.

Usually, the person who tells you he doesn't drink much water, will soon be telling you of his physical or emotional problems, sometimes, his allergies. Or perhaps he doesn't sleep well. He always tires easily. He may even be short-tempered.

Drink a glass of water before you do anything of importance. Drink a glass of water when you first get up, perhaps two.

Drink a glass of water at least once during the morning.
Drink a glass of water at least once during the afternoon.
Drink a glass of water sometime during the evening.

In addition, you will have other juices, beverages and soups. At the very least, liquids will dilute the poisons in your body that may affect your judgment. At best, they bring refreshment and cleansing. Don't forget them. You will find that the world looks brighter. And you will look brighter to the world.

4. *The importance of momentarily putting aside all stress.* A worried man simply cannot put aside his stress just because he would like to do so. It doesn't seem to him practical, or even honest, to let go of his anxieties, which are so pressingly important to him. But he can let them go for a minute or two. This does not offend his sense of responsibility.

Apply this advice to yourself. Close your eyes and say to yourself, "I am in control of myself enough to wipe my mind clear of stress for two minutes by the clock. Thus, I am not untrue to my duties. I can go back to my worrying in two minutes—but now, I let it go." You will find this surprisingly easy. You will be delighted with the feeling of success it brings. To manage one's own mind is a great feat.

You may have to argue with yourself a little to accomplish this command of your thinking the first time. But, you will find that it is really easy, especially if you say inwardly, "I could stand pain for two minutes. Certainly, I can manage my mind for that length of time to think of something agreeable!"

Exactly what happens in this brief time? Your nerves get a sudden, wonderful release. Your mind gets glimpses of more attractive sequences on which to focus. But the chief benefit lies in the success, however short-lived, of self-assertion, self-management. For two minutes, you are in the authoritative position over yourself! For two minutes, *energy*, the parent of all life, flows into you in various ways, to refresh your mind, body and your whole attitude.

In this two-minute holiday, a man gets a glimpse of his possible hold on himself. He senses the remarkable cooperation of natural forces that flow toward his demand, *if* that demand is in harmony with the laws of *life*. Consider what life really means —hope, growth, reach, newness, pattern, beauty, becoming, always becoming. Concern yourself with life if you want LIFE. Energy is LIFE.

Everything in the natural world works for you, never against you. Even in the teeth of disaster, a man can build anew and swiftly and better. The law of growth is ever at his side. Think of these laws and the feeling that you are slipping, losing, spent, that you are tired, or failing, will disappear. For life pours itself into every acceptance of it, just as electricity leaps into a conductor.

5. *The importance of moving the dead ashes of fatigue.* When a cell is born, there is a minute explosion of energy. It is a scientific fact that a cell, fed and kept cleansed of waste matter, can live "indefinitely." Its life possibility cannot even be measured.

When a cell dies, its small bit of "ash" joins the other waste matter in the body. All of this debris, this residue, must be moved out. The used-up materials of the body must be carried away from the healthy, clean tissues, if they are to live their wonderful, long life.

When you are tired, stiff, logy, it is partially because the dead ash of fatigue is not moving along as it should, to the organs of elimination, but is sluggishly polluting your system. To stir it up, and move it along, here is an exercise that you can take even while sitting at a desk in an office. I call this one "the invisible exercise," because you can take it without seeming to be doing anything.

The invisible exercise. Tense your body all over, beginning with your feet. Tense your legs, your thighs, your stomach, your chest, your neck. Hold yourself hard, Hard, HARD! Count six. Now, let go. Make your body soft as butter. Relax every muscle. Let the blood flow through every particle of yourself to carry off the "ashes" you have squeezed into a new position, where they will be picked up and carried to the organs of elimination. Repeat this squeezing and letting go three or four times.

In a few minutes you will feel a surge of new energy. Use this exercise at least twice a day.

Learn to rest sitting up, as well as lying down. You should learn this one for many reasons, for you can do it practically anywhere. It is not as easy as the others I have given you, but you will like it. It was taught me by a Hindu, Harendranath Maitra, a pupil and protege of Tagore. I call it—

The coat hanger exercise. You are going to hang up your body as though it were a coat. Your shoulders are your coat hanger. Your spine is the pole on which you will hang it. Naturally, the pole must be straight. Also—

YOU MUST LEARN TO SIT "ON BALANCE"

1. Starting at the chair seat, stack your vertebrae as though you were building a post of bricks, one on top of the other in perfect alignment.

2. Relax your hands and place one on each leg, as far forward as it is comfortable.

3. Sway slowly, slightly forward and back, then slightly from side to side, until you find the exact point of your balance. Your poise should be completely exact so that no muscles are used to hold you in position.

4. Now, draw your shoulders up, Up, UP under your ears. Hold them there while you count six.

5. Now, suddenly, forcibly, thrust your shoulders down as far as they will go. Hold them there firmly, tensely. Count six.

6. Now, turn your head from side to side slowly, tensely, chin over shoulder on each side. Six times.

7. Now, let go! Your head will be balanced on top of a straight spine. Your body will be literally hanging on your shoulders. No muscles whatever are being used.

Sit in this erect, but limp, position for two minutes. Gradually, extend the time to five minutes, or as long as you can devote to it. This is a wonderful exercise for everybody, but especially for those engaged in close mental work, or delicate precision work, or demanding calculations. Fliers use it with excellent effect. It is ideal for anyone who wants a real vacation from stress, but who has little or no time to spare.

Another way to quick refreshment is to brush your entire body with a dry brush. Your body has more surface than anything else. Your skin is a real barometer of your state of being. It shows, at once, if you are rested or fatigued. It is also an organ of elimination. It also breathes. Stimulate it. Keep it active, and it will add greatly to your well-being.

If you are an insomniac it is important to learn that you can get a great deal of rest and refreshment, without sleep, *if* your thoughts and emotions are gentle and pleasant. In any case, stop worrying about it. Do *not* take sleeping pills. (Let tranquilizers and benzedrines alone, too. You must master your own life.)

The one advance I want you to gain from this book, more than any other, is that you will take charge of your own life, your own body, and your own mind. Even if the pills for this and that are good, and harmless, they contribute nothing to your mastery of yourself, which is the purpose for your being here on this planet in any condition whatever! Your soul learns nothing from a pill, no matter how fine it may be. A false energy, and a false control—are just that—false!

Doctors are needed. It goes without saying that almost everybody needs a good doctor at some time in his life, and that the new medicines are wonderful in their best uses. But that does not refute the fact that too many people take too many pills. Dump yours out in the trash unless you are under a doctor's orders for some specific reason. Do not doctor yourself, but begin to reconstruct your energies.

When you take charge of yourself, you will be surprised how well your body will get along and improve. You will be astonished by its obedience when you mean what you say when you speak to it. These ideas will be developed later in the book.

These few suggestions in this chapter are for a quick effect, a needed "comeback" when you are tired but must go on to other activities. In order to keep our feet firmly on the ground instead of sailing off into nebulous notions, we must prove each step of the way we shall go. Now we shall set about the fascinating study of energy itself—and your having, or not having it.

4

⌒　⌒

YOUR EXCESS BAGGAGE

HOW TO RID YOURSELF OF EMOTIONAL BURDENS

Having now "conditioned" your mind and body not to accept the idea of fatigue, you must be alert to supply every prop and help to support your new "picture" of yourself.

You are a traveler through life, a guest at the inn, as Omar put it, therefore, you must look to your baggage. What are you carrying with you? Do you have excess baggage? How heavy it becomes! How expensive it can be!

A LESSON IN WEIGHT

Have you ever weighed in at an airport and been shocked by the amount of money you must pay for the excess weight you carry? Well, I remember repacking my bags in Frankfort, Germany, and shipping all but one back to Paris, while I took "Le Grand Tour." I learned, at that time, to travel with one suitcase plus a large handbag, thus relieving myself of excess charges, the heaviness to carry and the worry about it.

In repacking my bags in Frankfort, I discovered that most of the overweight was in things I did not really need, that the amount of personal effects I did need weighed about the allowed poundage on the ticket—a refreshing discovery!

Then, how had I accumulated the extra, expensive weight? Largely by not using good judgment in choosing between the important and the unimportant weights. So, let us ask ourselves—

WHAT ARE THE IMPORTANT MATTERS OF LIFE? THEY FALL UNDER
FOUR HEADINGS:

1. Health. 2. Faith. 3. Love (friendships). 4. Money (material advantages).

Why are material advantages put last? Because, without health and friendships, there will be no career and, thus, no money. They all tie in together. Then, whatever works against health and friendships works against happiness and satisfactions. Since all these "desirables" are on the salutary side of life, they have perforce, a common denominator, a welding, annealing factor.

The major base of all well-being is faith. By this is not meant a Sunday faith alone, but a day-to-day, work-a-day faith, one that is so strong, familiar and constant that it works automatically.

A faith in the basic rightness of the universe.

A faith in the goodness of life as it was meant to be lived.

A faith in the goodness of people, as they are allowed to develop their natural liking for all members of the human race.

People have to be taught to hate. They have to be propagandized and conditioned to it. But, however it is acquired, it is excess baggage, and therefore expensive.

Let us think of life as a current. When it flows naturally, uninterruptedly, it seems to bring, or create, lovely things, pleasant relations and extensions of man's creativity. But, whenever its flow is dammed, cut across by a delaying, inhibiting or stultifying moment or condition, its effect is blunted, garbled, misshaped.

This flow of life is like a beautiful agreement between motivating force and creative ideas. Like attracts like. Watching this process of constantly moving force and matter, in form or happenings, should teach us how we can emulate it, and use it to the benefit of mankind.

It is as though we were looking into a kaleidoscope of intricate patterns, each piece of which falls into its proper place, making a fascinating design. Move the glass, even slightly, to the right or left, and a new pattern will be formed.

We can form a new, lighter pattern of ourselves by putting aside the burdens of self-doubt, dislike, criticism and all their unwholesome ilk. (There are many who will defend these weeds of the mind as having certain values, and perhaps they have, but they are too costly and too messy for our new and better ways of going.) Some self-training is required before profitable facility is gained in choosing only things of value as mental baggage.

The entire universe is in movement. Every atom and every planet is constantly moving. *Ergo,* why not reach for a change for the better? Why should we cling to the same old short-comings, ailments, poor opinions of ourselves or anyone else, the old dullness, rejection, hurts—any and all of those emptying states that spell fatigue. Have done with them!

Repack your mental baggage. Do this for a lighter, swifter, more pleasant and profitable journey! Throw out everything that is not contributing handsomely to your welfare—old grudges, for instance. Some of us are straining every nerve to make good, just to "show" someone who may have spoken lightly of us long ago.

It is good to have some kind of spur, but isn't an ideal a bet-ter one (with no headache afterward) than vindictiveness. The trouble with trying to make a virtue of the proddings of anger, ego, inferiority and jealousy, is that even though they do spur an individual to great effort, there is a residue of emotional "poisons" that must be dealt with.

A man may make a fortune while lashed by one or all of them—then pay most of it out to psychiatrists, analysts and doctors and health spas to try to deal with the left-over tensions and tangles; his residue of "waste" is still dangerously radio-active and not presided over by government. Such a man usually thinks his condition is the fault of someone else, or that things went against him.

A CASE IN POINT

I remember my mother's trying to get a maid to clean her house more thoroughly than usual. The maid resisted all mother's gentle or subtle requests and suggestions. Finally, mother became so angry that she grabbed the scrub-bucket from the maid's hands, pushed her aside and knelt down to use the soapy brush in the corners. She cleaned the room as it had never been cleaned before and then, she slipped and fell, spraining her ankle.

She said to the girl, sharply, "See what *you* made me do!" Her back was hurt and she developed a headache besides. But, as she lay on her bed of pain, her ankle in a poultice propped on a pillow, she said quietly and truthfully, "No, I guess I can't blame my lack of control on that simple girl. If she had had my opportunities for education and social training, she might have developed more self-control than I showed. Take a lesson, Margery, no matter how much others may provoke us, the final decision as to how we will react comes from within ourselves." Brave, honest little mother! (She lived to be eighty-eight in perfect health.)

Later, she apologized to the girl. And, miracle of miracles— the maid began doing better.

AT ONE TIME OR ANOTHER, ALL OF US IMPEDE OUR OWN GROWTH AND FREEDOM BY BLAMING SOMETHING OR SOMEBODY ELSE FOR OUR UNHAPPY EXPERIENCES WHEN THE FACT IS, THAT OUR OWN INNER DISCORD CROPS OUT UNDER PRESSURE! IF WE WOULD LIGHTEN OUR LOAD AND ADD TO OUR STRENGTH WE MUST CONQUER INNER DISCORD

Just because somebody else supplies the stimulus to bring it out, doesn't mean that it isn't in us and very much our own! How could someone else "make" us angry if we had no anger to have?

Anger burns up the electrical wattage of our energy at a very fast rate. True, a madman has, temporarily, the strength of several people. Often it takes three or four other men to subdue him. Scientists can explain the exact process by which the madman's residual strength is telescoped into any given moment.

The measuring, discriminating, conscious mind has lost control. The glands, under the stimulus of rampant, wild ideas and intensified desires, pour their impulses and hormones into the tissues and bloodstream, multiplying the man's normal strength several times. It is as though a live wire had fallen in the street, misplaced, dangerous, destructively powerful.

The madman may sleep for twenty-four hours later, in an effort to recover his physical losses. But what of the less tangible losses, the destructive pattern impressed within him? These are matters that will require the best efforts of his psychiatrist to stimulate in the patient a desire for self-control. So-called normal people should measure their own burn-up of anger against this story. It is said truthfully that any comparison of normalcy and insanity is a "matter of degree, not of kind."

OVEREMPHASIS, EXAGGERATION, TOO MUCH FOCUS AT ANY POINT, SPILL ENERGY. THE TENDENCY TO GO TO EXTREMES IS EXPENSIVE, EXCESS BAGGAGE.

In a battle, in danger, especially to those we love, we call properly and normally, on our natural provision for greater strength. A human mother, or a tigress, trying to defend her young, shows astonishing strength and cleverness.

But these emergencies, even though they are prepared for by nature, are not the main part of our lives. It is the day-to-day victory over the "little foxes that spoil the vine" that counts in our favor. The little envies, the small constant resistances, the petty dislikes, these become walls, erected brick by brick, between us and the flow of our good to us. How heavy they become! How strangely people cling to them!

Do you carry excess baggage of petty dislikes? Does someone's habit of pressing his lips together annoy you? Does someone's voice "drive you crazy"? Do you "burn" inwardly when you are kept waiting by your wife (husband), or a business man whom you are trying to see? Do you curl up inside when you smell some hated aroma? If the answer is yes, you are doing a very strange thing,—

You claim to dislike these and many other things, yet you are enthroning them as matters of great importance! You are giving them life-giving attention, when the real way to kill anything is to ignore it, until it ceases to exist for you. You are carrying these dams, resistances and negativities with you, when you need the space for something of value! (If you want to remove something, do so, without burning up so much of your inner energy on the worthless matter.)

How often do you say, "I can't stand that shade of red" or "I *hate* that type of car" or "That fellow's personality rubs me the wrong way." Why don't you find something you *do* like, so that you can live affirmatively, *drawing energy?* When you hear someone gathering the weeds of conversation instead of its blooms, you might say—

Who appointed you judge of everything and everybody? Have you received any anointing from on high? Has an angel appeared in a dream to tell you that God appoints you to judge His world? Did you receive any telegram from the President or the Governor asking you to form an opinion and to report on anything imperfect that you may find? Unless you are paid handsomely, you will find devotion-to-whatever-is-wrong an expensive and a damaging hobby. It is expensive in many ways. Here are but three:

1. It keeps your mind off the bright and the right, which you need.
2. It prevents the flow of good to you and kills it on contact.
3. It estranges people and kills their faith in your loyalty. (See chapter on Friendship.)

THE LAWS OF LIFE OFFER YOU RELIEF, NEW ENERGY, NEW LIFE WHEN YOU MEET THEM ON THEIR TERMS (NOT YOURS)

If you were going to breed race-horses and race them for prizes and money, you would learn everything possible about every aspect of breeding and racing. You would keep every detrimental thing away from your horses and you would seek advantages in every way.

You would expect your jockey to be of certain weight so as

not to overburden your horse when he needed every shade of his strength to speed over the line ahead of the other horses. You would not say, "Well, I'll just put these rocks under the saddle this once and hope it won't matter," or *"My* horse can race with a hobble on, because that is the way I wish it to be."

Ridiculous as these remarks may seem to you now, they are no more ridiculous than that someone would expect energy and health while carrying the dead, useless weight of self-doubt and/or guilt. While these are the burdens of all ages, they are the ones most likely to be troubling the young. They haven't lived long enough to gather a mass of smaller, more subtle ones.

Self-doubt and guilt assail the young. But they cover up remarkably well with bravado. Wouldn't it be wonderful if youngsters could be taught that they are packing their emotional bags for a long trip? And that the contents of that bag may drag them down unbelievably, therefore, they would do well to keep it as light as possible?

The answer is not a loosening of standards so that they need not feel guilty in areas of self-indulgence and self-interest of many kinds. The best solution lies in giving them the strength, the vision and the courage to keep their standards high—and to bear with mature strength the sting of failure when they must face it. We are certainly not serving the best interests of progress to put our stamp of approval on behavior that means retrogression, instead of advance, for the human being in his reach for greater strength and higher power.

It is better to stumble toward an ideal than to pull it down to match imperfect performance. Instead, they should be taught how to face failure bravely, not suffering too much over the error, because they will have inwardly resolved to do their best toward more self-discipline.

Our young people are not relieved of guilt by telling them it is all right to behave like young animals in the woods. They have far too much sense, too much native intelligence, to take comfort from that false premise. Even though they pay lip-service to it and take full advantage of the looseness implied, their sharp minds would penetrate the misrepresentation and their inner burden would be just as great, and greater.

There is great comfort in the truth that controlled and appropriate behavior is the way to advancement for the whole human race. But also, young minds should understand that forgiveness is not a whim of a temperamental god or a detail of some particular religious teaching, but that it is a *principle* inherent in the basic law of survival, continuance. Just as nature equips us with the process of sudden strength under stress conditions to save our lives, she makes us also subject to a process called redemption, or healing which goes on whether we will or no.

The wound *heals,* (if we let it) the winds blow away the dry dust of error. The waves wash out footprints in the sands of time—and no man who loves life, respects his God, (whatever he conceives Him to be), and trusts the laws of the universe, need carry a burden of guilt forever. Let him accept the forgiveness, the healing which is part of his very being, as a merciful gift of the Creator and in gratitude live closer to the purpose of living at all—to progress, grow, evolve and discover his inner strength.

If we confess a misdeed to a human parent and receive his loving forgiveness and his support in our efforts to do better—how much more can we trust the love and the caring forgiveness of the great Creator of our whole universe! Put your guilt down, it is heavy, truly excess baggage!

To know that the Creator loved us enough to put that process here for us should certainly evoke our grateful praise and joy. Such love understood, begets our love, and a man acting under the law of gratitude and love can be trusted to give a good account of himself.

Nature did not intend you to carry a burden of guilt! But neither can you toss it aside in a cavalier fashion. Talk it out with someone, but be sure that someone is trained to listen to you, else you may be giving someone a hammer over your head. A trained analyst, a man of the church, these are your best recipients of your unburdening.

Accept forgiveness. Forgive yourself. Then you will more honestly forgive others, which is just as important. (For if you are holding the memory of an error, it is *yours,* no matter to whom it originally belonged!) Get rid of it.

Guilt, for any age, is exhausting. Everyone must find a way to deal with the normal amount of "guilt-feelings" that burden his life. They take many small and large revenges upon him. Guilt expresses in hundreds of ways. It reduces a man to a kind of slavery, for he must continually compensate for his low opinion of himself. Guilt colors one's entire outlook. It is like putting an ugly, colored slide between you and all you see. Everything you look at is tainted by its hue. A burden of guilt can be so heavy that it weighs down your whole life. One seeks, in many ways, to shift the weight. Probably, the most important word in this entire subject is—

COMPENSATION

The things one says and does to "make up for" his guilt-feelings!

One's ego may strive continually to make someone else pay for the discomfort he feels. One makes a fetish of finding other people at fault. It seems important to pull as many people as possible down to one's own size. One may even become foolishly generous to make himself feel better about some particular misdeed. (It is said that gangsters feel this urge and by large donations hope to "buy themselves some ice in the hereafter".)

One can be driven by guilt to try to excel and become worthy in some other field (one of its better products). One can also be driven to despair and loosen one's grip on life.

A large percentage of divorces can be laid to the inability of two people to get the demands of their separate guilts working together. How much energy is wasted in their running battle, for days, weeks or years!

THE BATTLE OF THE SEXES CAN BE A BATTLE OF GUILT-COMPENSATIONS

Down through time, writers have spoken of "the battle of the sexes," and "the battle of egos." But often the real cause of the battle is submerged—and its name is guilt. By freeing oneself and freeing others, one makes a sensible step toward strength and harmony.

A man who has really healed (not just ignored) his guilt-complex finds that most of his outer battles no longer exist. He is no longer "on the defensive." He is no longer "sensitive" and irritable. He gets along with people and doesn't read something offensive into an ordinary remark as he used to do. The short-circuit of inferiority is unsnarled and order now rests where all was fight and chaos before. He is poised, peaceful, objective, elegant. He is a victor and as such he can now afford to consider the other person a great deal more.

One of the chief things to guard against in dealing with one's guilt is the tendency to defend it. The sooner one admits (to himself, at least) his erroneous position, the sooner he can set about its solution, thus, free himself.

One need not have committed a murder to gather a sinking load of guilt, nor does it always come from a single fault or wrong. It is often built up from scraps of experiences, failures, embarrassments, small ways of falling short.

But there was a cornerstone laid somewhere in the past. It may have been a hurt, a loss or shame, perhaps something that might seem quite trivial now. Yet the sharpness of the emotion suffered at the time may remain just as acute, though buried, and may make one especially sensitive to fairly ordinary experiences.

It is usual to hold closely the blame one may have had originally for the person who was most responsible for the hurtful occasion. Some people have developed a callousness to enable them to carry the original hurt. Others have become progressively more sensitive to emotional pain. While the latter ones suffer more, they are more easily helped.

Why carry it around for a lifetime? Some people are still making their friends pay for the fact that away back in kindergarten, they gathered the hurt of rejection in a game or competition. One has to walk around their feelings as though one were walking around eggs.

Energy flows in when inferiority goes out. All the paralyzing, involved, grip of the machinery of inferiority collapses when one really understands that one has access to all the clean, fresh power that he can grasp. In fact, he can have a great deal of it, if he will just get his impeding, old, tenacious pictures of his wrongs out of the way.

This moment is fresh and new. Why bring the debris of the past into it! Why say, "I've always been this way. I'm unlucky. I always have these headaches on Wednesdays. I've always hated string beans. I can't stand jazz music. I don't like string quartets either. And I can't see any sense in ballet. I don't like to dance. I don't like cucumbers. My partner's wife is so difficult to talk to, she wears me out at a dinner or a party. I can't stand conversation at breakfast. The new manager of the foreign department gives me a pain. He thinks he's God's gift to women and really, he's just a drip. Now don't ask me to go to a movie starring Lawrence Olivier. If that's acting, I'm John Barrymore. This tax situation has got me down. I'd move to an island, but if I did, they'd start using it for bomb testing. Don't talk to me till I've had my coffee. I don't care if it is the only television that works, I want to see my ball games. No, the children can't have it for a half-hour, and you can't have it for Liberace either. Why do I have to say I love you? I married you didn't I? Anyway I told you last week. Don't forget to send my blue suit to the cleaner and what on earth have you done to your hair? It looks as though you'd combed it with an eggbeater. Yes, dear, you have lots of charm—I seem to remember. What did you do with my vitamins. I left them right here on my table—oh, here they are in my pocket. O, I must tell you I got a big kick today. You remember that Scott fellow who got my job with First National when I was just out of college. Well, he was up to our company today. The president called me in and said he'd given my name as a reference. I said to myself, "Now's your chance, after all these years, to get even with that so-and-so." But I didn't want to look mean. So I just kept my eyes on the floor and shrugged and said, "Maybe he's changed in all this time." I glanced at the president's face and saw I'd had the desired effect. Let me tell you that was a lot of satisfaction. Say, you know that pain keeps

coming back in my right side. Oh, that's stiff! Guess I'd better
go down to the Turkish bath, or stop and see Dr. Mead in the
morning. I'm not old enough to get these kinks, etc., etc."
(Would you care to diagnose this person's rapidly increasing
age?) I imagine one would have difficulty finding a constructive word or feeling in this speaker's whole day!

WHY WON'T WE LISTEN TO THOSE WHO TRY TO TEACH US?

Two thousand years ago, a Nazarene said, "Inasmuch as ye
have done it unto the least of these, ye have done it unto me."
One of his meanings was that the "Principle of Sonship" (the
Christ within) was the receiver of the offense of our thoughts
of our fellow men. I am a Christian, but the teachings are
simply those (in part) of the way things work in our minds and
interrelationships. One need not attach any religious interpretation to understand the fact that what you say or think of
someone else is truly your own, for the thought is brewed in
the secret places of your own mind where your ideas are born,
and you are in it and it is in you. We bear the shine or the scars
of our constant thinking. It could not be otherwise.

The Greek poet Pindar, five hundred years B.C. said
"Nothing aids the health as a peaceful and fair state of mind!"
Aristotle, who was thrown down stairs by his pupil, Alexander
the Great, probably said, "This sort of thing shakes my body
up, but it does not disturb the truths I teach you." No wonder
Alexander adored him! From Socrates to William James, almost all great thinkers have agreed the mind was far more a
deciding factor in our state of life and state of health than
any other.

Hippocrates (c. 450 B.C., the "father of medicine") thought
it was time people took the "treatment of the soul into account." Galen (of hygiene fame, second century A.D.) spoke
of how disturbed and low emotions could undo the good of
the finest care. There is certainly nothing new about this knowledge. What may be new, is that people have come to the point
where they are ready to train and discipline their thoughts and

feelings. We seem to be ready to separate the sheep from the goats in our own consciousness.

We have finally come to realize that no matter whose fault it is, ugliness in the mind and heart is *excess baggage*. So are self-doubt and excuses.

You are a child of the universe. Self-doubt is tantamount to doubt of the universe and the Great Mind that created and animates it. This is a kind of blasphemy. Clear the cobwebs out of your mental eyes and *see* that, as the highest of creatures on this planet, you have access to all the power you can understand and grasp.

You are a highly complicated, amazingly integrated being, and you possess capabilities as yet unrecognized. Make a brave start in believing your supremacy and *acting* as though you thought it were true.

GET YOUR THOUGHTS AND YOUR FEELINGS WORKING TOGETHER

Suppose one part of your "intellect" is saying "Yes I understand my being one of the highest creatures on this planet with many privileges and possibilities," and then in the next breath doubt is saying, "I'll be rejected as usual. I have about all I can expect of life, and that little may disappear. Besides I don't feel well. That old clammy feeling of failure is right with me." What do you think is going to happen?

SELF-DOUBT BELONGS TO THE EXPERIENCE OF THE IGNORANT PAST. SET IT DOWN

As everything is in movement, move your old ideas and dark feelings right out with the junk. Move out all sense of inferiority, guilt and self-doubt. Move in confidence, the serene aplomb of one who is fed from within from the well-spring of divine creativity. So solid is your footing, that you can afford to be calm and confident—and can afford an occasional failure without embarrassment. You are rich enough to be wrong!

The Light Touch

People who are not very advanced are the more violently expressive ones.

Leaders, rulers, those of personal power, are usually those of trained restraint. A show of public anger, if it reaches the violent, will often cost a man more "face" than anything his enemies can do. Prestige and respect go down as though attached to an electric dimmer when one "airs" his private ill-will and lack of control about anything. He may continue in power for a while, but the public have lost confidence in his serious opinions.

Even the little man wants the leadership he has to bow before to have public dignity. He doesn't want serious judgments to be mixed with uncontrolled passions. The violent man has numbered his own days. The screaming leaders shriek across the political sky and descend as though they were the tail of fireworks.

Even the small spites that actors once in a while show on television, cost them a great deal in public respect. We may continue to watch their programs for our own reasons, but the star has come down several notches, never to be elevated. The public has a long memory for poor character in those who are in higher positions.

When these matters arise in the entertainment world, causing little flurries of news and gossip, the sin is far blacker if the opponent is a woman. Real men know it is still a man's world and that women are supposed to enjoy their gallant protection. One would suppose that kind of thing to be dead, but the truth is that the demand for chivalry is still dangerously alive! A few men, who were basically unchivalrous in the first place, are sorrowfully waking up to that truth. It bears constant repetition.

UNATTRACTIVE, SELFISH, UNCONTROLLED EMOTIONS ARE HEAVY, EXCESS BAGGAGE

The price paid for them is often unbelievable. If one would travel upward rapidly one must have the "light touch" of smoothing over the error. People without finer feeling simply cannot take it in that society (association with other people) *is* (supposed to be) a pleasant place. And poor darlings, they keep screaming about their wrongs until no one cares any longer. With experienced, unselfish smoothness they could have gracefully discounted the whole matter, whatever it was, and emerged victorious as gentlemen.

Remember that wonderful line from *Candle in the Wind*, "Men and beasts have always fought—and men have *always* won!" How wonderful to be a real man!

THE DISTAFF SIDE OF CONTROLS

Part of a queen's training is to ignore whatever may happen that is wrong. And if one may not ignore it, then patch things up quickly and get back to pleasant matters. Lest one reject this principle as too flossy and only for the crowned head or the white-tie set, let us see at once that it is a deep-rooted rule of life itself. When the present Queen Elizabeth of England and Philip were in South Africa years ago, a reception was televised. Someone dropped a tray of dishes in the background. Most heads turned to see what was wrong. But the queen did not even move a muscle of her face. She kept looking away from the awkwardness and did not interrupt her conversation at all. Many people spoke of her control and how much they admired her for taking no notice of the embarrassing accident. Why wouldn't it be just as fine for all of us to ignore the error, to build on the virtues and to have control enough to do so?

If it is good for a queen, why would it not be good for all women? If that is considered the "highest" behavior, why should we deny it to ourselves? Is not royalty there, after all, to represent the highest we, in general, may reach; a symbol of our own best selves? In any case, we Americans can certainly benefit by some of the disciplines.

The highest we know is the ideal of ourselves! It is our *raison d'être*, (reason for being) toward which we grope from our animal state, from savagery to the "light touch."

Don't you admire the man or woman who can calm a child

with gentle musical laughter which communicates confidence? That same manner and sound can calm other discords, too. Harmony in our most intimate relationships, often hinges on our ability to smooth over the gauche, to soothe the hurt of embarrassment, to focus on something fine instead, all with the "light touch" of experience and the knowledge of our power to do so! Then we find we have little or no excess baggage.

5

~ ~

THERE IS A RIGHT AND A WRONG WAY TO RELAX

RELAX *INTO* AN AGREEABLE, CHOSEN STATE, NOT JUST *OUT* OF SOMETHING

Please read this chapter slowly and carefully for it is on a delicate subject and I do not want to be misunderstood or misquoted. Be sure you understand it before you apply it to yourself.

Pay no attention to people who tell you to relax, unless they tell you also, how to tense for action, and how to coordinate the two. Don't just *relax!* Gracious! You might stay that way, like the little boy who made faces at people. Pay no attention to careless talkers who tell you to let go of your tensions permanently. When you are dead, you will have no tensions as we know them. A corpse is, from our point of view, completely relaxed.

Extremes in anything are likely to be disastrous. I knew of a man in New York who held classes in "relaxation." His students were delighted, at first. It was fine to "let go" and "rest." But after several years of this procedure, four of my five friends who went to him, had relaxed right out of their marriages, their businesses, and two of them were dead. They had relaxed right out of their bodies!

Wise rest for those who need it is a must. It is public knowledge that part of the accepted treatment for certain heart trouble is bedrest. No sensible person would oppose the wisdom of this recommendation where it is truly advised by a doctor. If

45

he has told you to take this bedrest, you had better do so, and stay at it until he tells you that you may get up. Not only will strain be taken off your heart and your liver, but you will be removed summarily from the program of days in which you built up too great a load for your body, plus the anxieties that accompanied it.

This removal from the usual pressures and loads, will, barring complications, give your body a chance to restore its functions to normal, as the healing forces of nature flow through you to that end. For it is this urge of nature that rejoins the sides of an incision, strengthens weak tissues and repairs any part of the body. No doctor has, as yet, learned how to do that. It is a mystery of life.

The life-force within you is always working for you. It is always building, healing, protecting, reusing the material at hand in miraculous fashion. All it needs is a chance. It is astonishing how few people get their mental and emotional debris out of its path.

Their petty discord, resentments, hurts, held as though they were important and precious, build up into real blocks to the natural flow of healing power. These people are standing in their own light. How quickly healing takes place when we get our emotional junk out of nature's path! If relaxing accomplished this kind of house cleaning, it would serve far better than it does. But relaxing usually does not solve a problem at all, it just temporarily ignores it, which may have a slight value. But it is misleading, because most people think that relaxation is going to cure them—of everything. It doesn't.

Many people who are trying to learn to relax need a doctor or a psychiatrist. The fetish of relaxation has delayed real help all too often. Now, let us back up and examine this whole idea again. Nature uses a fine *combination* of tension and relaxation in her finest structure, the heart. To subscribe to either relaxation or tension without the other is to throw nature's best plan out of balance.

Life is movement; movement requires tension. How is that fact expressed in your body? You have a wonderful muscle in your chest cavity that is active from the moment it begins to function before birth to the instant of death. That remarkable muscle is in your heart. How does it keep going, going, going for many, many years? Watch it closely. Observe exactly how it works. It tenses and then relaxes, for a split second, tenses, relaxes. Thus, it can go on, and on, and on. There is a tremendous lesson for us here.

The lesson of the frequent rest, Nature's best way. An experiment in fatigue at Columbia University illustrates the point. A tiny, lead weight was tied to a man's finger, as his arm lay on a table, before which he was seated. The object was to discover how many times he could raise that forefinger before it was exhausted. Working with a metronome, he lifted the tiny weight thousands and thousands of times. Finally, his finger was completely paralyzed. He did not recover the use of it for several days.

With another man the experiment was made another way. He was to lift the weight for two counts, and then pause one count, lift for two counts, pause one count. The man could continue this type of action as long as he could stay awake!

THE VALUE OF THE FREQUENT REST OPENS AN AREA THAT SHOULD BE CONSIDERED BY EVERYONE

And is it not reasonable? Life is expression, articulation. Each idea appears to create or draw the energy for its expression. Apparently the birth of an idea, as the birth of a cell is a tiny explosion—a fresh impetus. The stream of life, then, is a series of what might be termed pulsating motivations. In any flow of energy, such as electric currents, there are billions of separate impulses.* It is not the steady, unbroken flow it appears to be. The lesson is clear—the pulsing of the heart, the pulsing electric current. They are not, of course identical, but you will observe that in each there is a sequence of actions. So, it would appear that we are somewhat in line with the way nature expresses herself when we follow with a series of movements and the frequent rest.

---

* ". . . Einstein postulated that all forms of radiant energy—light, heat, X-rays—actually travelled through space in separate and discontinuous quanta." *The Universe and Dr. Einstein,* by Lincoln Barrett.

A trip during which I grew more rested instead of tired. I applied this principle of periodic spending of energy, during an automobile trip across the country several years ago. I was at the moment my little story opens, lecturing in Denver, and I had made an appointment in Des Moines, over seven hundred miles away, with a publisher. I had also made a mistake in my calculations. I had to stay on the road to get there in time.

Why didn't I telephone and make another appointment? Because the man I wanted to see was leaving that day by plane, to start on a trip to Europe.

I remembered the theory of the frequent rest. I would drive for two hours, then stop and sleep for twenty minutes in the car. I would draw to one side in a "service area" off the turnpike at two-hour intervals and ask an attendant to call me when the time was up. After several of these pauses,—

I found that I could "set" my own mind to wake me. The mysteries of our possible mastery of the entire self are worth our most serious thought.

By the time I had reached Des Moines, with a half-hour to spare, I was more rested than when I had left Denver. When I arrived in New York, my friends thought I had had a vacation, I appeared so refreshed and bright-eyed! By using the frequent rest in many ways and places, I found that I could keep myself refreshed and ready for many extra hours of activity.

I DISCOVERED THAT I COULD PREVENT MYSELF FROM GETTING TIRED

This subject is worth a whole chapter of its own. Many people will have to adapt this practice to the demands of their busy lives.

It would be quite impossible for businesses to operate for a two-hour period and then stop for twenty minutes! But, individuals can avail themselves of some of the suggestions I have given and will give throughout the book. If business men would adopt them, we would not lose so many of our best executives at age fifty-five.

Thomas Edison used the frequent rest. We are all familiar

with the story that he required only three or four hours of sleep. A closer scrutiny of his habits will show that he dozed from time to time. He would close his eyes and lean his head forward or back, slip off into a nap, a very short nap. Perhaps this frequent contact with the sea of *mind* called "subconscious," gave him some of its secrets when his conscious mind was asleep. I have been told he also took short naps lying down.

It pays to keep refreshed. I had an uncle, a very successful man, healthy, well-adjusted and rich. He always took a nap right after lunch for ten minutes. He used to laugh and say that he made most of his best deals in the afternoon when other men were sagging and he was alert. Action—relaxation! And now here is one of the most important ideas to be considered—

Do not relax out *of a situation. Relax* into *one.* Thus, you will be staying in nature's pattern of always moving forward, ahead. Examine your feelings and motives when you are tired. Nine times out of ten you will be wanting to get away—and this negative approach to a perfectly normal action will spoil it for you.

Always go *toward* something. Go toward rest, refreshment and new action. Put your thoughts on these aspects of leaving work. Don't just resist the situation in which you find yourself.

At first glance this choice of motive seems too subtle to matter, but it is very important. A longer study of it shows it to be the difference between a *dynamic* approach and a *deadening* one. It does seem strange that two men can do exactly the same thing, but, from such a widely different premise that they will get almost opposite results from the act.

Consider the fact that the universe is always moving forward. There are no backward looks in all of nature, so far as we know. Apparently, creative nature is not *repelling* anything to even half the extent that she is being *drawn to* something. We can do no better than to study nature's ways. Relax *into* something. You can even wax poetic and think of relaxing into "the arms of the Infinite" (Trine). As you let go, mentally and bodily, do not think of how tired you are. Think of how pleasant it is to pause in order to think how rested and fine you *will* feel. In this way, you are *agreeing* with the way the life-force seems to work. Perhaps this is one way to apply the Biblical injunction, "Agree with thine adversary quickly— lest . . . deliver thee to the judge." Perhaps the adversary is the negative approach and the judge is the law that seems to bring a punishing result when we do not choose a constructive way each time we have the privilege of a choice.

Relax constructively. Do not just "fall apart" and think how "gone" you are. There is a way to make almost all of our thoughts and feelings constructive.

WE SHOULD MAKE CHOICES BECAUSE WE *LIKE* SOMETHING, *PREFER* SOMETHING, AND NOT BECAUSE WE DISLIKE OR ARE REPELLED, REVOLTED BY SOMETHING

If you take your tiredness and your worries with you and mull them over when you should be directing your attention gently into pleasant, refreshing ways, you will "wake up as tired as when you went to bed." How often have you said that! Remember that negativity is the short-circuit that drains your power.

Remember that constructive choices multiply energy. When you relax, let go of every thought of fatigue. Fall back into a dynamic state of pleasantness, into that current of power by which nature runs and rules her universe. Let it suffuse you. Let it flow into every smallest part of you, bringing its perfect pattern into you. Think quietly and gently of some pleasant project ahead.

All your choices should be dynamic, with no rejection in them whatever. If you turn in distaste from the weariness of your job, you will find something distasteful in the next job, and the next. You will have turned your mind to the "distasteful," and where your mind is, your experiences follow. That is the law, the inexorable law, that is fulfilled "to the last jot and tittle." I do not mean that every single thought bears fruit. But it certainly contributes its weight, and colors the atmosphere of your life.

Remember that the right relaxation is a preparation for action. Otherwise, it is nonsense and has no real point. It is not a negative blotting out. It is a positive preparation.

6

THE RIGHT TENSION

TENSION IS NECESSARY TO EVERY THOUGHT AND ACT

The very words "tension" and "attention" are derived from a common root meaning "directed aim or focus." Then why has the word "tension" come into such disrepute. Tension is important to us. The tension in a violin string gives it tone and quality. It is important to all continuity of action or thought. We cannot live without it. We cannot breathe, move or think without it!

There is nothing wrong with tension, as such. But *why* are you tense? In your answer to that question will lie the reason why it is good, or bad for you. Being tense about wrong ideas and feelings can kill you. Being tense about good and happy plans attracts energy, thus, more *life.*

It is bad for you to be tense through fear of failure, loss of affection, loss of attention, or loss of your job, or prestige—or fear of being late and looked upon as an irresponsible person.

What is the motive behind your tensions? Are you tense with hate—old hate or new hate? Collectors of hates usually have both kinds. (And they tell you what and whom they *don't like* endlessly!) These tensions cut off the flow of life-force (which is, at base, approval, love and energy) and will wither your body as well as your career and your hopes.

If you are tense in joyful anticipation of some gala event, or intent upon some fascinating work, discovery or game, you will draw energy to yourself. If you are bright-eyed and eager over the idea of buying a boat and picture yourself sailing it, fishing from it, and entertaining your friends on it, your blood

51

will be coursing happily through your body carrying messages of alertness and pleasure. If you are thrilled over getting ready, dressing meticulously to go dining and dancing with some especially admired person, then your tension alerts and electrifies all the salutary processes in your entire self.

If your tensions make you tired it is because you have the wrong ones! And sometimes a very tired person is deeply tired of himself; he may even deeply dislike himself.

It is said that, under analysis, Cary Grant, the handsome, highly successful, though no-longer-young, romantic leading man, discovered that he hated himself and was "taking it out" on those nearest him. Finding it very difficult to get along with people, he stayed away from them to preserve the romantic image.

After he was shown the reasons for his hostility, his suspicions, fears and wrong tensions, he became as he is now—gregarious, hospitable, generous, loving, and happier than he has ever been. But the chief result of the mighty release of his long held negativity is that he seems to have recovered his youth! His joy brings back what Carl Sandburg has called the "juices of youth" and he is as active and playful as a colt in bluegrass. It is like being born again to get rid of the debris of years!

The right tensions restore youth. Unhappy tensions are the greatest enemies of young tissues and attitudes. Youth want to *do* things—to dance, to climb, to go somewhere, to make something, to project wonderful plans and to share with friends and loved ones. Youth is full of fine tensions that both attract and create energy.

Douglas Fairbanks, senior, whose energy was prodigious, used to break off rehearsals, but instead of resting in a chair, would go into some athletic dare or contest with members of the cast and crew. In a few minutes he would come back full of zest and crackling with new ideas. He used to say, "When every fence you pass doesn't dare you to jump it, you're getting old!"

Most of us have no desire to jump fences, that is, those made of wood or concrete. But we ought to get very excited about jumping the emotional fences that hem in our lives, stifle our laughter or creativity, and drain our strength.

Get up the steam of enthusiasm about dealing with those barriers. Develop a happy tension over that project. And you will find it more than profitable.

You'll never get over a wall of any kind in a state of unhappy tension—or a state of relaxation! (Both these conditions are unproductive.) Energy truly does not come from resting. Activity of the right kind, the right tension, actually creates energy. A dynamo is a machine of action. It creates, or collects, a force called electricity. It accomplishes its purpose by *movement,* not by relaxation.

Los Angeles is a sprawling, growing series of communities. More power is needed constantly to light and to service these extending areas. When a new subdivision is to be opened, do the managers call the electric company, and say, *"Rest* your dynamos. We need more light." Certainly not! They knew that the dynamos must run extra hours to make extra electricity, or more of them must be put into action, or some other method must be used to bring more power to the new community. But it is all *action.*

The next time you think you are dead tired, don't try to rest. Drink a glass of water. Eat an apple. Go for a half-mile walk, maybe farther. You'll be refreshed and good for three or four more hours work, or play. That is, unless you took your unhappy tensions with you. Forget them, having trained your mind to do what you tell it to do.

Note the small details about you as you walk. Be aware of the sound of laughter, a snatch of music, the flight of a bird, a long shadow lining a tree. Give yourself over to the right "attentions" too. Beauty creates energy!

RIGHT TENSIONS GIVE YOU ENERGY—
THE WRONG TENSIONS ARE ROBBERS

I have had the experience, time and again, of feeling more energy at the end of a day than at the beginning. At certain times, I teach (interview) all morning, have a class in the afternoon, tuck in one or two more interviews, and have another two-hour class in the evening. (Since I was young, people have come to me for advice on social and domestic problems, for private training in the amenities, and to help them coordinate their best points. In late years people have sought my spiritual and philosophic counsel. I am happy to share my wide experience of the world and living. As, in a sense, a Guru, they sometimes come and stay with me.)

Over and over people say to me, "How can you stand that grind? Aren't you simply dead?" It is impossible to convince people (whose minds are closed) that I have *gathered* energy instead of *expending* it. Sometimes, in Los Angeles, I get out and walk for a half-hour at the end of such a day and evening, to "walk off" my charge of energy in order to go to sleep.

What could be more energizing than to see people walk away from your counsel light-hearted, freed of their burdens? What could make you feel more powerful than to see a roomful of "tired" people gradually come to life as they receive your dynamic truths about the way they *can* function. When they entered, they sank into their chairs in little heaps, and started dutifully to listen. Then, bit by bit, they became convinced that the Author of their being had not meant them to be dragged out by a day's work. They started to straighten up. Color came to their cheeks. Chests and heads lifted. Eyes snapped with the brightness of fresh ideas and new impetus.

They told me, with great sincerity, as they filed out, how grateful they were for the facts and the feelings I gave them. They went out joyful, triumphant, laughing. Of course, I felt like Mrs. Hercules! I felt one with the very force that moves the worlds!

WHENEVER AND WHEREVER WE TOUCH THE PRINCIPLE OF ENERGY, IT FLOWS INTO US

The comparatively little energy I had spent in talking, standing and thinking was a drop in the bucket when compared with this dynamic inflow from the fountainhead of all power! Experiencing this gain again and again over many years, I have come to know that *the principle of energy is life,* never its opposite. I realized that my own puny strength hardly mattered. Energy was a principle I could touch. And when I touched it, I was one with it. It was mine!

7

⧡

ENERGIZING YOUR MIND

AS WITH A HOUSE, ONE FIRST CLEANSES, ELIMINATES,
THEN FURNISHES FOR FINER FUNCTIONING

THE FIRST WAY STARTS WITH A MATERIAL POINT OF VIEW

1. Look over the site, take note of the available materials
   and build your building to fit the situation as you find it.
   This way is considered very practical by careful, unimaginative people. There is a certain amount of good
   old-fashioned common sense in "cutting the garment to
   fit the cloth."

(If a man wanted to embark on a certain adventure, he most
certainly would not plan to do more than he could support
with supplies and materials.)

But there is another way to fulfill a purpose.

THE SECOND WAY BEGINS WITH A VISION OF THE IDEAL

2. Make your plan. Draw it on paper. Make it wonderful—
   make it ideal. Put in all those fine new ideas that have
   glowed like bulbs of light in your mind. See your structure (a house, a career, a service, or whatever) as an
   extension of yourself. Create it on paper, exactly as you
   wish it to be.

PUT YOUR FAITH BACK OF YOUR IDEAL PLAN

Know that only men who dare to plan beyond the practical
materials on hand at any given moment have ever given much

to the world. Edison dreamed of light and bridged the way to it. When space is conquered, it will be a dream which drew its fulfillment! (The "practical" people always talk against innovations.) A truly dynamic idea draws power to itself that somehow finds the materials and the means of its fulfillment.

RESPECT YOUR IDEAS

A good, careful, average success can be based on the practicalities of the issue, but the striking discoveries, the new departures, the reaching designs and revolutionizing plans begin with the *idea. Then* consider the subject of how you are going to get your materials. Never be too willing to settle for the materials around you. Suppose you lived in a community near a sandstone quarry. You need not confine yourself to sandstone for your building. You can, if your imagination and demand are sufficiently bright and strong, bring marble from across the world for your structure. You can have papers and hangings made to your own design at home, or you can order them from India, China, England, Africa, or anywhere.

LET YOUR MIND SOAR, ENVISION, DREAM, AND DEMAND

Let the world be your front yard. Dream your own dream and let no space or border hem you in. Live in your world and *use* it. Let its largeness expand your soul and pour its energy into you!

A DREAM IS A NUCLEUS

As the song from *South Pacific* goes, "If you don't have a dream, how you gonna have a dream come true?" And as the lovers in du Maurier's *Peter Ibbetson* said (and sang, since Deems Taylor made an opera of it), "Dream True," that is, live your dream until it becomes real.

Never accept a limiting thought, thus, you will more surely build your *inner demand* for more and more energy. It is well to cultivate largeness in every way. One may not be small in some ways and large in others without running the risk of being small when one wants to be large.

Dare to make your plan a fine one. Do not abandon it. Learn to be patient. Thinking of the perfect plan instead of local or limited materials often forces one to find ways to make the seemingly mediocre, familiar materials serve so differently and elegantly that they take on a glamor they never had before.

RE-EVALUATE YOUR PRESENT STATUS

I had a friend whose house began to be a little shabby. The whole place looked—well, tired. She couldn't make up her mind just how she wanted to improve it. She decided that she wanted all new furniture. But she delayed and delayed. Finally, she called in an excellent decorator, a man brimful of new ideas. She felt her whole life would hinge on the different slant she was taking toward her house. Her husband finally agreed to let her do as she chose about it.

A clean sweep, she felt, was needed. She wanted to throw everything away and start afresh. Her husband could not really afford such an extravagance; there was quite an investment in the furniture on hand. But he held his peace.

As the decorator became immersed in the problems of her house, he began to value first one piece of furniture and then another. He would say, "This chest is 'good' basically. Its lines are satisfying. The color is wrong, only the color. This chair is lovely. It needs a stripping and a new velvet cushion."

By bringing in entirely new ideas on the uses of the rooms, planning striking wall treatments, and painting a few pieces in the open rooms on the first floor a very soft coral color, the whole appearance of the place became unified, elegant, dramatic—and far more comfortable than before.

In the end, most of the old pieces were used. Everyone was astonished that in their new dress and new placement and use, not only were they adequate, but they made the rooms very beautiful. And so it is with most of us. The things we have gathered into our minds and lives have far more value than we now recognize or enjoy. A masterly, knowing plan can reinterpret, re-use, re-color, and replace to advantage the material of our past. But we must be willing to accept the new interpretation and let the dead wood go.

CLINGING TO USELESS, OLD WAYS OF DOING THINGS DRAINS AWAY MENTAL STRENGTH

Try to be objective, not emotional, in weeding out the useless and salvaging real values. Don't try to cling in sentiment to old things and habits and at the same time attempt to benefit by the new ones. Whatever you keep from the past must fit into your new pattern, your new interpretation of yourself.

LET GO! IT IS EXPENSIVE TO BE LOOKING FORWARD AND BACKWARD AT THE SAME TIME, LIKE THE TWO-FACED GOD, JANUS (FROM WHOM WE GET THE WORD "JANUARY")

There is a widow whose deceased husband was a very remarkable and charming man. They were an unusually happy couple during his lifetime. And now that he has been gone almost fifteen years, she is still living in the happy marriage they had. She should marry again. But the few men who have interested her grow fearful that they cannot measure up to the enshrined ideal in her mind. She is still a widow.

Her friends occasionally bring a new man into her circle of acquaintances. The new man is invariably attracted to the very presentable and entertaining widow. He takes her out two or three times—and then, no more. He gets tired of hearing about so much happiness in the past when he wants to put a shine on the future.

DO NOT CLING TO THE PAST—EVEN A GOOD ONE!

Again, we should take nature as a guide. The past (as we have noted) interests her not at all. Observe again the struggle man makes to preserve the relics of the past for sentiment and information. Nature attacks the cohesions of time gone by and works steadily toward their obliteration. Whatever her reasons for this tearing down process, she also has more vivid and vigorous pressures toward creation.

SHOW ME SOMEONE WHO LIVES IN THE PAST, EVEN A HAPPY ONE, AND I WILL SHOW YOU SOMEONE WHO IS GETTING VERY TIRED

To prove this point to yourself, just listen—that is all, just listen. This man, or woman, is becoming exhausted, and may contract a wasting disease—indeed, may already have it.

Be careful that *you* do not try to bring too much of the past along with you. Suppose you are having a beautiful marriage, and have several lovely children. You might then say to me, "Do you expect me to brush out of my mind the happy memories, the high happiness, the soaring pride that have been mine in all these years? In the pages of my memory are pictures of thousands of situations in which we were all happy to be together, to see the children grow. How dear they are to me! These memories are my life. I cannot do without them."

NOW LET ME GIVE YOU A LITTLE MENTAL TECHNIQUE THAT WILL PERMIT YOU TO KEEP THESE MEMORIES WITHOUT HARM

I repeat: no matter how happy your past, if you live in it, you are asking for nature's disintegration! "But," you say, "my past is so wonderful, I must bring it along." You may, but in this way only:

1. Form a mental picture of yourself as a person who is the product of a wonderful past, a great experience. Bring the focus up to date.

2. Think of how the past has contributed to your present richness. See yourself as a person of rich experience who has been blessed in many ways.

3. Think gratefully of all you *have,* not *had.* If you focus on *had* you can lose what you *have.* (If you do, you will have asked for it.)

4. Look ahead to the many years you will have to enjoy what you *are* because of the experiences you have had.

ENERGY DOES NOT RUN BACKWARD

Energy, as a principle of nature, moves only forward. We cannot use it for ourselves in any way that is contrary to its laws. We cannot expect to hold energy, which moves forward, if we are thinking backward.

WE BECOME LIKE THAT WHICH WE CONTEMPLATE

If your mind is focused on thoughts and matters that are synonymous with disintegration, you will become immersed in the pattern of decay. It is easy to observe the way this action works in other's lives. It is more difficult to see it in ourselves. But, as we have already said—

Never turn from anything in distaste or revulsion. Turn toward that which is new, fresh, and desirable. But also bring the *values* of the past with you.

A proper sentiment (in homeopathic doses) about your own past is poetic, pretty, and pleasurable. But do not bring with you for too long a time either the good or bad aspects of former days. Sorry, but nature is interested only in the new moment, the thing or creature now being created.

A woman carrying an embryo in her womb learns that if she doesn't supply the materials for the growth of the fetus, nature will take what it needs from other parts of her body. One recalls the old saying, "Every new baby costs the mother one tooth, at least." It is certainly true that if the expectant mother does not furnish lime and calcium enough for the new baby's bones and teeth, the life-creating process going on within her body will take those materials from the handiest place—*her* teeth!

The new chance, the fresh start, the clean slate, these seem to be the obsessions of nature. She seems to be aiming in a determined, if somewhat blind, way toward improvement. Why do we not study her and take the lessons she can teach?

I am an advocate of sentiment and the precious values of a life well-lived, with all its fine moments and memories. I am, however, pointing to the fact that we had better put such things in their proper place—and not let them usurp the throne of first importance in our lives.

There are, of course, lessons we have learned through our own past experiences and those of other people. They fill our histories. We should value our former experiences and hold the more useful and valid parts of our inheritances.

We should not divide our energies by trying to live in the present and the past. We want to know history for many reasons, but chiefly that we may improve upon it in the future of the human race. Too much looking backward (unless one is an archeologist) is destructive and will destroy anyone who indulges in it overmuch.

IF YOU WANT MORE ENERGY, LIFE, YOU WILL HAVE TO GET IT FROM THE ONLY SOURCE, THE FORWARD LOOK AND FLOW: THE CREATING, BECOMING, SHAPING LAW OF THE UNIVERSE

You can help gather energy in your mind by having projects. Look ahead. Have concrete plans, for the living, not the dead. Actually envision your future. You may change these plans and visions, but have them you must. Something from the creative force within you must reach out toward the future if you want to become *one* with the flow of *life.* Your entire mind is energized in the process.

HAVE VISIBLE EVIDENCE OF YOUR PLAN

If you do not now have the money for the plans that intrigue you, work with them anyway, on paper. Have one of those amusing banks (pigs) marked "My trip to India," "My new factory," "Our swimming pool," or whatever. It is not probable that you can get money enough into that pig for a new factory. But the project is re-stated every time you look at the thing!

Reiteration creates a nucleus about which other forces and matter gather. Do not be too proud to use the repetitive theme to help you in your aims. Use everything! Energy flows into clear ideas. Repetition brings clarity.

We Must Articulate Order and Clear Outline in Our Thinking

Set aside a time every day when you will restate silently your new ideas and goals. Remember, you must displace the old, useless, damaging ones with fine, bright, new ones. Take at least five minutes several times during the day to envision your desired objective. *See* yourself in possession of the experience. You energize your ideas by reiterating them and by visualizing them.

Call Your Determination Into Action

You will have to be faithful in holding to your new mental patterns. A wispy wish or two will not make much of a ripple. It is the constant drop that wears away a stone. You are making entirely new paths in your "gray matter."

Are you willing to be patient while you add, add, add the strength and brightness that will replace the old unwanted patterns? It takes some doing! There will be times when your vision will dim and you will wonder if you are working in the right way. These are the times to cling to principle. Reason yourself again into an acceptance of the truth that all begins in mind and work again from that premise.

There are times when you must say, "Here I stand, faced rightly on the path of creativity—and here I *stay* until I prove my point." Do not waver, but tighten your thinking around the truth you know and watch the law of mind work.

It is by using your mind that you sharpen its edge. Give it *extra* things to do, to learn, if you want to energize it. Resting your mind accomplishes nothing but its softening. Keep it taut, sure. It is the person with a tight schedule who can always make room for one more duty or favor. The loose thinker can scarcely get through his own little day. Get the negative debris out of your mind and demand more action of it!

Theodore Roosevelt was a great advocate of the idea that a change of pace is an energizing vacation, and it is surprising how many great men have espoused that practice. When your mind is "tired" from columns of figures or wrestling with knotty problems of any kind, don't try to rest it by not using it, or just by thinking how exhausted you are making the poor thing. The cure for that kind of mental fatigue is to ask your mind to do something quite different. The thing most highly recommended for this "change" is to memorize some poetry. Such a revolutionary idea for a man or woman with a tired mind! One can almost hear the protests; but don't be like Mrs. Patrick Campbell "firing on her rescuers." Try it! The proof of the pudding, you know.

The next time you think you are mentally fatigued, learn a verse by heart. It is surprising how many an octogenarian is a poetry spouter. Prick your oldsters' minds and find out! My mother at eighty-seven could recite for two hours without stopping—and she was always learning new poems. Now what could be the connection between poetry memorizing and a long life? There *does* seem to be one. Let's examine it.

1. Poetry has the singing rhythm of the tides, the accuracies of mathematics, the demands of soothing music, the balances of equations. It sets up this basic, lulling consonance with the way the world runs, and thus "plugs one's mind in" to the strong rhythmic currents that support the whole.

2. One of the mind's mysteries is its ability to remember. This delicate process of recalling is dried off like unwatered tendrils on a plant if not used, and especially if denied. (Most of us are always denying our memories.) If we put our negations aside and tell our memories what to do, they usually obey. Remembering poetry seems far easier than recalling prose, probably because the very lilt demands something like itself and only a few words *could* come next and since the choice is limited, the most appropriate one suggests itself. Yes, we become enmeshed in a whole fabric of salutary reactions when learning poetry. The whole matter becomes a cushion for life's rougher buffetings.

3. A person with a mind full of tender, amusing, or epic poetry is almost never lonely. He escapes that most cankerous of all human afflications—loneliness. Wherever he is, he can draw up into consciousness some apt quatrain and occupy himself with the remarkable word-picture some great poet left for us. This companioning by the great nourishes the heart, truly gives it surcease and balm—so why wouldn't it last longer than one torn by unrelieved stresses? The very words, "learn by heart" are truly chosen, for unless the verses fall deep into the "feeling" nature, they will not be retained. Remember, in Proverbs, "As a man thinketh in his heart, so is he."

LIVING IN THE GREAT SEA OF MIND, STRUGGLE IS NOT ALWAYS THE WAY TO ACCOMPLISHMENT

Often, after we have established good habits of effort and response, we can do faster, finer work by ceasing all conscious effort and inviting the inflow of native intelligence. Sometimes our finest thought, our best ideas, *float* into our minds. Therefore, we would do well to have quiet periods.

MANY PEOPLE BELIEVE THAT GENIUS IS BUT A FULLER FLOW OF MIND WITHOUT MUCH EFFORT

This may be true, but genius seems to rest more surely on those who have put in a great deal of work, trained their muscles and reflexes in whatever art or process is involved and thus invited, prepared the way, in a sense earned, the higher way—as though it were the overdrive in an automobile.

Swifter, higher, keener ways are open to everybody if each person would sweep out of his mental path the debris of lower thinking. Many talented people let envy kill their careers by sullying their inspiration. Clean up your mind and keep it clean!

We have discussed the weight, the excess baggage of envy, hates, grudges, and hurts. Who among us does not bear their taint to some degree? Still, many of us feel almost weepy and sentimental about our hurts. We cling to them.

ARE YOU CARRYING A HURT

I knew a truly angelic woman (in every other way) who never forgave her father for forcing her to some unimportant decision. She cherished a rancor on the subject for some forty years! It colored her whole life. So sensitized had she become to the idea of someone's dictating to her that she would not even accept a suggestion from a well-meaning friend. Her husband was punished most severely by her smarting ego. She became a virtual "dictator" in her house, all because she was afraid of someone's "ruling" her life. Naturally, she was a semi-invalid.

Probably every teen-ager passes through this phase of suffering ego, but a grown-up is supposed to have resolved such tangles and arrived at a mature vision of give and take.

PEOPLE WHO REMAIN SO HIGHLY SENSITIZED TOWARD AUTHORITY ARE CASES OF ARRESTED DEVELOPMENT. THEY ARE STILL TEEN-AGERS, NO MATTER WHAT THEIR YEARS

We have observed the unbelievable expense of a grudge. One would suppose we had long since outgrown such immature nonsense. But have we? What unbecoming things we do when we have a grudge! Look in the mirror when joy leaves your own face and a feeling of envy or enmity steels your soul. It is as though a searing, burning desert wind has passed over a bed of flowers and left them an ugly tangle of withered stems.

DO NOT MAKE YOUR ENEMY SO IMPORTANT THAT YOU GIVE HIM POWER TO SPOIL YOUR LIFE

You need only a few hours of *grudging* to starve your brain of the vital forces it needs and gets when your emotions are comfortable ones. Why not have your glands exuding energy (salutary hormones) into your body instead of poisons? It is not just that your face will look better and finer. Your deeper feelings affect your deeper organs. Why not have energizing hormones passing into your blood stream and that stream, in turn, flowing fresh and unhampered into your brain?

THE THINGS WE DO TO OURSELVES BECAUSE
SOMEBODY ELSE DISPLEASES US!

If the person against whom you may have a grudge knew or understood the effect of it on your own body, mind, and life, he would probably be delighted. When we truly mature emotionally, we will put aside all such worthless procedures. Worthless? Dangerous! Why will we waste any time whatever on such things when the whole world lies before us as a great gift from God! How generously it responds to our slightest obedience to its laws.

WHEN SORROW COMES

I walk gently into the subject of the effect of sorrow. The law is the same—but pity and understanding soften our words. We can only stand holding out a hand to anyone in the grip of sorrow. Overwhelming loss leaves one inundated, breathing in its drowning sense of emptiness. One then must walk in that painful void with little vision of even a pale hope of surcease. One cannot say to a friend in this agony, "But this is wrong. You must not do this. It is bad for you!" Your words would probably fall on ears already numb, mercifully, with pain, while only your loving presence means anything. The words mean absolutely nothing.

But the very love for the one who is gone, the quality of love in the soul, slowly asserts its own gentle balm. Slowly we come to know that our finite understanding cannot encompass the intricate movements of the master mind and we finally find ways in which the strong brightness of *life* reasserts itself.

Though in the deep valley of grief we may not even wish to live, we finally come to see that it is not ours to judge, and that we will be better by trying to live as the one we have lost would want us to live. Not to be solved by a few bright words, our problem of loss gradually distills its own defenses and brings its own strengths in its own time. Be patient and gentle with yourself. Be gentle and patient with others. Time is not too important.

RENOIR'S "THE RIVER"

There was a beautiful book made into a beautiful motion picture by Renoir (son of the great painter) called "The River." It was a simple almost uneventful story of life in India by the river, the great Ganges.

The word "India" is from a root-word meaning "river," the current and waters of life. The story followed a young girl and concerned her moods and reactions, her beliefs and her acceptances—and they were gentle, with all the remarkable strength and resilience of acquiescence. She accepted life. She loved its many tender gifts of moving beauty, its small delights, its deeper grandeur. I don't remember the plot. Only the enchantment of the ineffable grace and graciousness of her almost melodic acceptance of life stays in my mind as a lingering perfume, for it seemed to be so in hers.

A FLOWING MOVEMENT WITHOUT STRESS

There was action, with no striving. While the story was conceived in the atmosphere of Eastern religion, it seemed almost a picturing of the Twenty-Third Psalm, "He leadeth me beside still waters. He restoreth my soul." In many ways, the philosophies of India underline the great and deep themes of the Occidental teachings. There is only one truth—and whoever has found it, by whatever means, East and West, has found his God.

THE TIMELESS BALM OF PURE BEING

The seeming effortlessness that comes of obedience to life's laws as rivers run to the sea! Then why the battle? Is it not born in man's lack of faith in his world and in himself? His answer may well be to get very still, beside some flowing stream, and try to know himself a part of all life. If he can *accept* the laws of his being and in that acceptance, obey, thus becoming master, he may have learned the lesson he came on this planet to learn.

I shall reiterate many times that we waste too much energy disliking things: certain people, certain ideas of politics, religion, *et al.* We are not required to approve of or embrace that which is contrary to our own best aims and patterns.

We should turn toward that which we like instead of from that which we dislike. We have not the privilege of condemning anything. It is presumptuous and arrogant. "Judgment is mine, saith the Lord." It is ours to prefer, to choose, not to criticize and condemn. Condemnation clogs our lines of energy.

NATURE IS ALWAYS RE-USING HER MATERIALS, NOT CONDEMNING THEM

Our own words show our acceptance of this basic idea. When a man leaves a life of waste and prodigality, we say he has *"reformed."* He is the same man. He has simply poured his energies into forms of living more in consonance with the seeming purposes of civilized practices (the greatest good to the greatest number).

APPROACHING LIFE ARTFULLY

Having learned some of the techniques of living well, we find we can shape most of the seemingly formless materials. When a man knows how to take a chisel, a hammer, and a piece of granite and, with a series of blows upon the rock, shape it into a form of beauty, we call him a sculptor. Yet each of us is shaping the *formless* every moment of our lives.

When a man takes color, canvas, and brushes and paints a lovely object, person, or scene in certain poses or views, we call him an artist. Yet each of us is arranging colors and taking positions that are harmonious or discordant all the time.

When a man artfully arranges the juxtaposition of notes and their sounds to cause them to express his feelings or to tell the listener a sort of story, we call him a composer, a musician. Yet each of us is creating pleasant or unpleasant sounds every time we speak.

Life is an art—we are constantly shaping it for ourselves.

Life is energy—we are using it to shape our own expression of it. We will choose and create what is useful, beautiful, and worthy. Anything else is nonsense.

Does it not follow that if we mold our inner patterns toward those of eternal harmony and rightness that we will then share, to some degree, the forces and qualities of eternal principle? Why would anyone waste his time and lose his way choosing inharmony, excess, lower themes, and the lesser, weaker way at any point?

ONE NEED NOT BE WICKED TO LOSE HIS WAY

One may be almost a saint and still miss the point. If a good man *believes* in the law of diminishment, he will have less and less—and find himself spent. If a man observes nature and sees that the more she spends the more she has, he can leave the path of diminishment and take the path of richness.

THE LAW HE ACCEPTS BECOMES HIS LAW

He believes that since recorded history and before, men have spent their energies and died; therefore, he must do the same thing. Saints and sages and his own inner voice may tell him that he need not do so, but he will not even hear them!

If he *expects* to be tired at thirty-five, retired at fifty-five, going at half-mast at sixty-five, slowed to a crawl at seventy-five, hardly moving at eighty-five, and gone somewhere around that time, he will act out the manuscript he has written for himself. The diseases he will get in order to carry out this "accepted" program will make it all very logical. Even *he* will never know that it was he, himself, who set the sequence of events in motion to carry out his sovereign demand, *i.e.,* the age-old "habits" of man.

WHY NOT BACK UP AND TAKE A NEW VIEW?
RE-USE THE MATERIALS AT HAND

You have within yourself, at this exact moment, all that you need to make, remake, or make again and again your expression of this stream of consciousness you call your life.

There is energy enough in your little fingernail to run a great city for several years! But you will never find it and learn how to use it if you have given your remarkable mind over to fatigue.

At this moment, probably nobody knows how to find and use it. But if we do not turn our minds toward it, we will never find it. One thing we do know beyond a shadow of doubt, man's use of his world begins in his mind.

REFORM YOUR IDEAS OF YOURSELF AND YOUR POTENTIAL; RE-USE YOUR ATTITUDES

When Elisha helped the poverty-stricken widow he asked her, "What have you in the house?" She had a small amount of oil. Beginning with what she had, he re-used it and created all she needed. This is one of the great lessons of the Bible.

Whenever you need anything say to yourself, "What have I in the house?" There will be some talent, some value, some service you can render, something you can create. Anyone who is alive is in touch with the great allness of mind and some evidence of it in him or around him can be multiplied to meet his need.

It is not necessary to go anywhere, or find something or somebody new. What you now have in yourself and your environment is as potentially divine as anything else. Act upon that divinity, lay hold of it, claim it, articulate it—and *use it*.

YOU CAN NEVER BE WITHOUT THE DIVINE POTENTIAL WITHIN YOU

We need not say, "Lo, here—" or "lo, there——" but look within. You can not "run out" of energy, for it is the very essence of your being, and of the entire universe. You *can* shut your eyes to it, accept the vegetable-animal estimate of yourself and become another sheep among the billions who are treading the path of diminishment.

And when you have acted out your accepted pattern, you will, no doubt, have a nice, respectable funeral, with the proper amount of tears, music, friends and flowers. Down through the ages, we have developed this weird celebration of our failure to understand *life*. It is nice that we comfort one another. It is a small, but sweet, compensation.

I hasten to state that I, Margery Wilson, am too much a

product of the tyrannical past to conquer fully this heritage of habits of diminishment. But I can make some inroads upon it and leave my findings for those who come after me. Knowing that all begins in mind, I simply hope to make a small crack in the general acceptance of the path downhill and urge us all to claim now an extra abundance of energy.

REINTERPRET YOUR ENDURANCE

See how much you can claim and how far you can go. To reinterpret the materials of your life is to start with an idea. To permit the materials to dictate the new forms is to limit the outcome. Looking first to the material side, one might just be tempted to settle for far less than is possible for him. Elisha, by his demonstration with oil, was trying to prove to the woman that her salvation from poverty lay not so much in the material, as in her *view* of it and *use* of it.

What have you in the house? A talent, or whatever, is merely your focal point, the channel by which your understanding of abundance can work for you.

Your view of your possibilities should always be ahead of your presently available materials. For instance, if you begin to think your energy limited to the strength in your food, or a nap, however fine and comfortable these may be, you will be forever a slave to them. One should do everything possible to build up his idea and feeling of strength, but having done them all, he must still know that he must rule his little world from within himself.

DO NOT GIVE OVER THE LEADERSHIP OF YOURSELF TO ANY MATERIAL THING OR PRACTICE

Use everything, but hold the reins yourself. Use and re-use your materials. Often a mere rearrangement of one's habits releases more energy. It is refreshing to prove yourself master of them. It is also very inspiring. As you feel your skills develop in dealing with your materials, you begin to be pleased with your growing power. You automatically think of still other ways to use them. This brings out the many subtle advantages of putting the world of *mind* before the world of *material*. One or the other will be master in our lives. One is expanding and the other is limiting. By treating material as the servant of mind we elevate it and multiply its uses.

Energized by mind, vision, pattern, faith, almost any material becomes the tool of new wealth, joy, accomplishment, or whatever. Take the familiar life you lead now, your family, your work, your house, and energize them with bright new interpretations. Admire, agree, rearrange your thought of them, and watch them become lifted in all ways.

THUS YOUR OWN MIND IS UNBELIEVABLY ENERGIZED.

8

ENERGY IS YOURS—BY RIGHT!

EVERYTHING AROUND YOU, IN YOU, AND IN THE ENTIRE UNIVERSE IS COMPOSED OF ENERGY

Yes, you have a right to energy. It is your legal heritage. You will not be trying to get something *extra* when you employ the means to energize yourself.

Energy is not a benefit you will wrest from a source opposed to your native right. Emerson, one of the greatest thinkers of all time, said, "The universe lies in smiling repose, waiting for the mind of man to act upon it." You may have as much as you learn how to encompass and use. This is true for *you*, no matter how tired, ill, old or spent you seem to be.

I say "seem" advisedly, for our sense of perception, all too often, receives and reports to the brain the wrong impression. You cannot trust your eyes, for instance, in all matters.

*Our senses are not reliable.** Your mind has learned to correct many of the impressions the eyes give.

1. In a motion picture, the wheels of a moving vehicle appear to be turning backward. Your mind must correct that report.

2. The sun appears to move around the earth. One can look at it and SEE it rising in the East and setting in the West. But

---

* "It is not surprising . . . that the prime mysteries of nature dwell in those realms farthest removed from sense-imprisoned man, nor that science, unable to describe the extremes of reality in the homely metaphors of classical physics, should content itself with noting such *mathematical relationships* as may be revealed."—*The Universe and Dr. Einstein* by Lincoln Barnett.

we have learned that this is not the case. Our minds must correct that *seeming* journey of the sun with the knowledge that it is the earth that moves around the sun!

3. Across the room, a round table appears to be an oval. An artist must paint an oval table if he is recording his visual impression. (And, of course, the world is not flat. It is not even perfectly round. Also, its orbit is oval, not round.)

In many instances, especially now, as our scientific knowledge is growing so rapidly, we must understand the TWO aspects of much that we see. (*Two?* There are four—or more!) There is the apparent and the real.

Mind only can know truth. Our wonderful senses, so necessary to our lives, must step down in importance. They are not the final judge of the truth about anything! Truth usually lies outside and beyond the realm of sense. Facts come to us only through the mind.

Understanding, concept, thought: these are the only way to emancipation of our erstwhile ignorant slavery to sense and the seeming. We are now after TRUTH that will make man aware of a larger share of the wonders of his world. *The truth is that man is many times more wonderful than he SEEMS to be.*

Man appears to be spending himself. But, as the song from "Porgy and Bess" says, "It ain't necessarily so." Man has accepted a now-universal concept of himself as a creature living out a brief story of *diminishing returns*—and when the last drop is spilled, or dried, he dies. Again "It ain't necessarily so."

Even Omar Khayyám, the dissolute philosopher-poet of Persia, penetrated the seeming drama of diminishment with his famous:

> Think then, you are today what yesterday
> You were—Tomorrow you shall not be less.

The fact of YOU, the potential of YOU is not lessened or changed by any mistaken idea or use of it. It simply remains a dormant, unused possibility, in the greater part. No less a thinker than Socrates said:

Something cannot emerge from nothing, neither
can something resolve itself into nothing!

(Oddly enough, these are the words that convinced me of immortality.)

No matter how broad these implications were meant to be, we can take some courage and new vision from them in the details of our living. For whatever is true on one plane of being is true at all levels. It remains for us to catch the glimpse of light that flashed through the mind of a poet or a philosopher—*and make it our own*. We shall keep out of some argumentative discussion, which may waste our time, if we stay with the broader areas.

There are even two schools of thought about whether the universe is wearing itself out, or gaining in size and energy. Einstein tended toward the latter view. It is the eternal argument between friction and cohesion—*i.e.*, friction wears away versus friction develops *attraction* and draws particles endlessly to its nucleus.

But, I assure you, it is not necessary to follow or understand the scientific basis of energy, in order to avail yourself of much of it. For in essence one finds it extremely simple to grasp.

Everything we can see, feel or think is an expression of energy. You are an expression of energy. Every particle of you is composed of it. You are also a vessel, a channel, for energy. You were born with enough of it to impel you through birth to childhood, from youth to maturity.

Then it is as though mother nature had said to you, "With the mind I have given you, by now, you are supposed to have learned how to take charge of your own supply. Now you are on your own. Not cut off from the parent, but honored by the power of choice, logic and discovery, you are now responsible for using intelligently and consciously the ALLNESS that produced you. If you do not take over, I shall have to deal with you as with other creations rooted in material mechanics. I shall have to plow you under. It is up to you."

Even a child can understand this. A twelve-year-old once said to me, "It is as though we had brought a box-lunch to the picnic—one packed by our mother—but when we grow up, we have eaten it and *must find our own food.*"

Natural procedure is not cruel. This perfectly natural procedure is neither a punishment nor any type of cruelty. There are people who say thoughtlessly, "Nature is so impersonal, so cruel." A closer study of the way nature has spread her riches before mankind makes us know that she is, at base, extremely kind, generous and providential.

Nature has paid us a compliment in supposing that we have the will and the good sense to make good use of her riches. Her laws are stretched before us, laws that, properly understood and operated, will give us more than we need of energy—and of everything else. "It is the Father's good pleasure to give you the kingdom!" Why do we not lay firm hold on more of it? Is it because we are too deeply enmeshed in the fatigues and limitations imposed upon us by the accepted, respectable reports of the senses?

I invite you to throw overboard the sense-testimony that you are tired—in any way—in any part. You have inherited, in the very air you breathe, the strength, the impetus, the thrust, to carry you much farther than you dare dream. But you must recognize your favorable, honored position. You must claim it.

Look at the world around you. You see everywhere strength, strength, STRENGTH. Worlds whirl through space, as far as the eye can see, and millions, billions of miles farther. They are both expending and attracting force—for *they are force.*

At the heart of matter lies the electron, a spark of volitional (within limits) power. There is no such thing as "solid" matter. All is energy, and energy is intelligent force—Mind. It animates all that is animate.

All growing things reach, without ceasing, toward the sun. A slender, delicate root will grow through or around anything that impedes it, sometimes splitting a rock.

The universal urge to be, to do, to express, is in you, in every fibre of you. Every living creature is in touch, at some point, with this movement of Life itself, else it could not be alive at all. To be alive is to be in contact with the life-force. And apparently, the amount of LIFE that flows into you and me is determined by our own capacity—our own individual inner pattern. The scope of your *pattern* describes the amount of life-force you draw and express.

You have a right to all the energy you can claim. If you are not pleased with the strength you now have, begin to change your inner concept of it. Alter that inner pattern of claim!

When you want more light from a lamp, you simply exchange the smaller electric bulb for a larger one, thus making a larger "claim" on the great supply back of it. There is no quarrel with logical procedure. It is the only way to get more light.

When you want more electrical power for appliances, you may have to put in heavier wires and other appartus to bring additional power for the service to you house. It requires a further investment to install this larger equipment, but it is the only way to get *more power* to run your appliances.

If a house stays in darkness, is swept with a broom, does not have any of the time and labor-saving conveniences or pleasures powered by electricity, it cannot be said that this is its "nature" —that it MUST be without power. At any moment of decision electricity could be brought in.

Power *is!* It exists all around us, on all planes. It is not "natural" for you to be without it, no matter how logically you can explain its absence. If you have less than you need or want, it is because the size of your intake is smaller than your requirement—and you are the only one who can correct the matter. It remains for you to find the way to command more of the great supply that was *put here for you.* It is natural for man to explore, discover and use his powers. But adjust the size of your intake to your need. If you accept a pattern of limitation, a cycle of diminishment, this is the sure way you will function!

Your pattern of claim and acceptance rules your life. There is no sense in berating a little bulb for not giving more light. *Change it!*

Life often seems to challenge us by surrounding us with temptations to deny our sovereignty. We seem hemmed in, burdened, trapped. But there is no situation where some of the laws of light and love cannot be active.

A PEDDLER WITH A GREAT SECRET

When I was a child, an Armenian peddler came to our door with a huge case of linens and embroideries. He was a small man and the case looked much too large for him to carry. As he opened it in our living room, the members of the household oh'd and ah'd over the exquisite contents. We bought a number of his wonderful things. We children were fascinated by the way he almost caressed the beautiful cloths and scarves. His great soft brown eyes seem to caress them too. We watched how magically he packed so great a number of things in that one bag. We hated to see him go.

We children followed him along the street to other neighbors and finally to the railroad station, marvelling with each step over the way the little man could carry his great load. Finally, we could bear our curiosity no longer and asked him. "How can you carry that huge, heavy bag around all day?" We seemed to sense that he had some supply of energy that we could not see.

The peddler smiled. A light came into his beautiful eyes and he answered proudly, "I am strong because my burden is beautiful!" Miraculously, we understood him!

The train puffed and huffed and smoked and took our new-found wonder out of our sight—but not out of our lives. To this day, when my burdens get heavy for me, I can see, in my mind's eye, the little man, kneeling before his case, folding with appreciative fingers the lovely linens, embroidery and lace as he packed them safely for the next move. We knew with what pride he would get them out for the next customer.

I can see again the pleasure in his face, the pride in his voice as he said, "I am strong because my burden is beautiful." And I have said to myself, "See to it that your own burden is beautiful, and you can carry it."

I knew that I had to weed out all ugliness and see only inspiriting beauty. When we think we are tired and spent, it is because we cannot find a shred of beauty in what we are doing or the problem we face. But *beauty is always present*. It has many faces. Often we must hunt for it—but "seek and ye shall find." At least, we can turn our minds from the stark demands that tire us and feel the worth of it as it restores order, gives some service or furthers some good end. Far better that we think of this than to sit mulling over our struggles and stewing in the whys and wherefores of our limp state. This is a foolish procedure.

There is no time or place when we cannot focus on worth and beauty. If we value our health and happiness we had better try to do so. If you have worked until two o'clock in the morning, what is to be gained by shuddering at the smoked-filled room, the mountainous ashtrays, the litter on the floor; or at how lonely and cold will be the road home, how annoyed will be your family, how short will be your sleep—and how tired you will be during the next day.

It costs no more to put your mind on how easily the room can be restored to order, how constructively you can use the time driving or riding home (you might even write a jingle to refresh yourself), how helpful will be the work you have done—and how wonderful to get it done! Have a little fun challenging yourself to be as fresh next day when you get back to work as you would be were you eighteen. You know you wouldn't feel it at all. Think of how marvellously good the bed will feel as you stretch out and sleep for five or six wonderful, restoring hours. How blessed you are to have such comforts! Actually you can draw so much that is good into your being by thinking rightly instead of wrongly that you can even improve your health instead of hurting it with dismal pictures that, like crows, produce after their kind!

You have the choice of hurting or helping yourself! Just working nobly, "killing yourself" as you put it, is doing just exactly that. Since you can call the turns why don't you call good ones?

The Question Arises—Why Is There Strength in Beauty?

Is it not because it is perfection of a sort—an accuracy—a realization of some height of pattern, being or doing?

Our minds hunger for it, as our bodies hunger for food. The

soul is fed and satisfied by beauty of any kind. "Man cannot live by bread alone." (This quotation is found in both the Old and the New Testament several times.) Beauty is the closest approach to the ideal that we know. Therefore we yearn toward it, seek to catch and hold it in art, strive to create it.

A great percentage of the world's business efforts are to gather and sell the appurtenances of beauty in some form. Ships ply the seas, raw materials are sought in jungle, desert and mountain to bring to milady something that will enhance her beauty or pay homage to it. Gigantic strength is expended in making and moving trifles to heighten the effect of her clothing, to adorn her house, to bring her pleasure.

The most exquisite building in the world, the Taj Mahal, was built in memory of a lovely woman. Artists who have caught on canvas some moment of exquisite beauty in a telling way find their works soaring in value. The masters today draw fabulous sums of money.

Singers who touch some inner chord of that yearning for beauty deep within us fill the great music halls of the world, and we cherish their memory when they are gone. Poets, who in the rhythms of words have given us back our highest thoughts, live in our hearts, and we revere them.

Why do we hold in high esteem all people who have reached a peak in their ability to reproduce, to express and to share with us the finest things the world has to offer? Is it not because as we find some inner identity with their works, our own strife and emptiness are appeased, emptied and forgotten—and our burdens are consequently lighter?

Why do we educate our young to be familiar with the writings and the creations of wise and wonderful philosophers and artists of the past? Is it not to give them pride and hope for the future of mankind—to encourage them to cherish and to follow their own inner higher voices that call them toward the beauty of perfection? Is it not because we know, however dimly, that perceptions of beauty will lighten any man's load? For ugliness and dullness are heavy, while beauty and rhythms of exactitude and harmony bring us consonance and rest.

These yearnings are deep in our natures. While education

helps to bring them out, there are many uneducated people who love beautiful paintings, sculpture, and music of the finest kind. Through it they find a contact with largeness that lifts them out of their small, immediate selves.

Beauty, perfection, rightness, and harmony are aspects of a principle in our universe that is available to every man. Its companioning, nourishing strength becomes for us the best kind of vacation.

A visit to a museum, a concert, or musical show might well bring more refreshment than an expensive trip to a vacation resort *if* the latter held the same old struggles, bickering and sense of inadequacy that one *may* have at home. We do indeed improve through relief from ugliness of all kinds.

To lift from any human heart its weight of error and self-depreciation is the goal of all art, from Rembrandt to our modern comedians. Laughter is a surcease from heaviness. Melody is a confection of soothing emotion. Dancing gives us the feeling of lightness, beauty and control, with the added joy of sharing it.

All the lovely things of life remind us of our higher possibilities and, therefore, give us deep, abiding pleasure. At such times we are in touch with fulfillment and companioned by the great ideal from which we spring. This is the pristine state of health, the true Garden of Eden, which, homesick, the soul is always searching to find again.

"But suppose my country went to war," a friend said to me, "is it possible to keep hate, fear and inharmony out of our minds when we are fighting an enemy?" My answer to that is that we can try—that we had better try. One can do one's utmost patriotically, and perhaps with more precision and efficiency, if he keeps hate out of his heart as much as possible. He will certainly last longer.

I seldom go to press without quoting a line given to Caesar in George Bernard Shaw's "Caesar and Cleopatra." Caesar is in Egypt incognito and meets the sixteen-year old Cleopatra who marvels over his world-wide successes. She envisions his power and his victories. Her eyes are gleaming, her breath coming in excited gusts. Finally, she almost shouts "Don't you just love to kill?" Caesar recoils from her with a faint shudder of revulsion and says quietly, "No, of course not. I just hold them, so they can't hurt me."

Another example I sometimes use is the one of the mad dog. One would not try to reason with a rabies-maddened dog terrorizing a community and about to attack some child. One would shoot, and as quickly as possible. One would not be thinking of hate. One would simply have the job of cleaning up a dangerous and messy situation. One doesn't hate a mad dog, but one must get rid of him somehow.

However desirable may be a world sans war—and one day we shall have it—it would appear to be somewhat in the future. God grant that we may learn to settle our differences at a conference table, and no doubt we shall, one day, do just that. But as long as large numbers of people are still barbaric, still animalistically violent, we may have to meet them on their level, hoping for the future a more civilized settlement of differences. The distant (but perhaps not vastly so) hope of the world is education, ideals, self-discipline, law, order and standards that are commonly understood. Certainly any organizations that stand for these ideals are going to be unpopular with the brigand-minded. But if we keep trying, the while defending ourselves as and when necessary, we shall have acquitted ourselves well in the pages of history.

I am not in a position to judge a man who tries to protect himself against barbaric aggression, or to aid, in honor, a friend to whom he has pledged his assistance. These are matters for wiser people in the ways of the world than I.

My advice is to the individual seeking to find the best ways of identifying and using the potential strengths within himself for a better and a longer life. He will find blessings for himself that he can share with others wherever he finds himself. Man's mistakes or brutality in no way erase his divine potential. One day we will all be civilized.

The Bible in several places predicts a world without war, tears or pain. We must be patient and faithful in working toward it, for it is surely coming. I do not believe that it is a great way off. This is a time of vision, growth and discovery!

Someday man's love of contest and power will be spent on training himself—a herculean task—out of animal bondage into a world of harmony and beauty. That will require all the strength he can possibly muster. He will develop skills, arts, find even greater powers, wipe disease off the earth, travel where he will, how he will—and evil will be forgotten. This is not even a religious prophecy, but simply an extension, in time, of man's necessity and his potential.

Meanwhile, he must meet the hates he has brought on his own head, solve the problems he has compounded in his ignorance and slavery to self and sense, and heal and advance himself in spiritual attainment. A very large order!

As we have said, art is a step toward the ideal. Even the neurotic picturings of discord are a record that the artist thought was worthwhile. He has a right to make them, to show forth his struggles with truth and values as he sees them. I am in the position, in that area, of Voltaire, who said to a man whose every utterance was contrary to his own, "I heartily disagree with all you say—but I will defend unto the death your right to say it!" There is value in everything. Through some of these art creations, those who come after us may know how bitter was our struggle, and therefore how great and shining may be our victory!

Beauty and accuracy are synonymous in many ways. The synchronizing of music and movement must be accurate to be beautiful. A painting that gives us a clear idea well stated, is accuracy. A motor that purrs in beautiful, smooth mechanics is a masterpiece of accuracy. The instruments of science that demand the finest exactitude are basically akin to the demands of music which are, basically, accuracy.

All machines of coordinated parts have kinship with a symphony orchestra wherein the perfect and unselfed performance of each part gives the magnificent whole. Anyone who has ever shot a gun or an arrow knows that he must rivet his attention on his target. He holds his sight on the bulls-eye, knowing that every fibre of his body will obey his demand upon it and will make the necessary moves, take the necessary positions (without specific conscious direction) to insure an excellent aim

Another way the response of matter to mind can be studied!

There is vast energy in the rightness of accuracy. Inaccuracy is very tiring. If you want to rest, then cure some of your inferiority by doing something extremely well—accurately, fully, without cutting corners or plotting to get away. STUDY THE ACCURACY OF THE MOVEMENT OF HEAVENLY BODIES. Strive for more accuracy yourself. Power will pour into you as you strive to do the RIGHT thing.

HOW CAN WE BEST USE THIS PRINCIPLE OF VITAL ACCURACY IN OUR LIVING? HERE ARE THREE WAYS

1. Seek accuracy in two areas: in work and in play.
2. Develop one or more skills, mental and physical.
3. Develop a talent.

One does not become a virtuoso overnight. At first glance it would seem that you are being asked to expend energy rather than to gain it. But there is no escaping the truth that one must invest in life before he collect dividends.

Energy flows toward the process of planting and reaping. You furnish the effort of ground preparation and planting, and nature will reward you with a harvest "pressed down and running over until there shall be no vessels to contain it." So natural is power that in it you live, move and have your being.

9

⟳ ⟳

PREPARING ONESELF
FOR SOCIAL OBLIGATIONS

SUCCESS IN SOCIAL LIFE, BY SHEER "EXTENSION" DRAWS ADDED ENERGY

This is the area in which our reputations are made. Our careers may demand most of our available energy, but it is the extra demand of social activity that often decides our standing with our fellow men. It is here that we are more fully vulnerable to other peoples' estimation.

A barrage of secretaries and inter-com systems may protect a business person from people during business hours, but in a drawing room, dining room or ballroom, or the local square dance, our more personal virtues, or lack of them, become apparent.

THE CHALLENGES OF LEISURE HOURS

Great and small men endear themselves to their fellows, or fail to do so, while the scrub women have taken over the offices. Their contracts, deals and blueprints that may spell glory will not help them a bit now.

Perhaps this is one reason why some men shun all social activities, and why others, perhaps busier, more influential men, enjoy getting out among people. One little secret of a person's preference along this line is the undeniable truth that

We like to do whatever we do well. But if we feel we are at a disadvantage socially, we pretend we do not like to meet others in this way. Though we may secretly yearn for some graces of the sort. (Many people are much too withdrawn. They tire! Every closed area dams up energy.)

It seems to be true that most "big" men learn somewhere along the line how to present themselves attractively in social activities. Almost all our "captains of industry" give a good account of themselves at a party or public gathering. Perhaps, earlier, at some pain to themselves, they have forced themselves to learn somewhat the ways and words of the social world—and then they seem really to enjoy it.

THE BROADER LIFE

Then they find that their social ease and success add glamor and recognition to their other talents. Life does indeed broaden for any man (or woman) who has learned how to greet people, to make pleasant conversation and to handle his body in an acceptable way. That does not seem to be too much to expect, but there are still some men who deny themselves and their families this kind of pleasure and profit. "What has this sort of thing to do with my success?" a man may ask. "I'm tired when I come home from work. I don't want to talk to anybody. I want to loosen my collar, and sit down in front of the television." Fine. Fine, that is, if his wife doesn't mind being consigned to a "silent world," with no one to share her thoughts and experiences, and unable to share his. No good life can be confined merely to one's home, no matter how large it is. A law of life is operating here, and that law says, "The more you withdraw, the faster you die." It's the same road—out! Why travel it?

Judgment must always be used. No woman should expect a busy husband to go-go-go all the time. But any man with an out-going mind should develop a desire to meet his fellows in the warm, cheerful, mannerly and well-presented life of gatherings outside his home.

No, a man's personal attention must reach into the community, his nearby schools, colleges, charities and other people's houses. He MUST if his life is to expand! It is a "human" obligation, since man is basically a gregarious animal. His community needs his smiling, loving interest. His presence is needed at his club, at his church and in civic matters. Civilization cannot go forward at its best without him. So he must find the energy to do his part—*after* his day's work, and after his helping and playing with his children.

Take a few minutes to "change gears." No one will deny him a ten-minute respite when he comes home. Let him lie down for those minutes flat on his back, on the hard surface we recommended. He will have disciplined his mind to the simple needs of young and old around him. He will talk and he will listen graciously to the hopes and claims of his children, and especially to his wife. Many a woman has been turned into a remarkable person by a husband who learned how to feed her life's needs when he came home.

A MAN WILL FIND THE ENERGY TO CONTINUE AS A MEMBER OF THE HUMAN RACE AFTER FIVE O'CLOCK

He will have trained himself to find pleasure in considering other people. And he will find that *energy follows pleasure.* If he dreads the claims of the evening, family and friends, he will simply grow *more tired* than he thought he was. For fatigue is a kind of accommodating accomplice to the don't-want-to theme.

A person can rationalize along this line until he really believes it himself. He can persist in self-education until a peculiar kind of logic backs up his determination not to go out and give a poor account of himself—so he'll just stay at home and do that! In self-defense, he must have "real" reasons for his chosen program. Then his body, having no alternative, will, on his demand, (conscious or unconscious) furnish them to him. He becomes ill in some way. Really ill!

SLOWLY, BUT SURELY, OUR BODIES DO WHAT WE DEMAND OF THEM

If a man has accepted the popular "dead-at-five-o'clock" disease, he will find himself a victim of it, a genuine victim. By following the practices outlined in this book, he can become a man of happy energy at any time of day. While he is a victim, he truly should not overtax himself just to be kind. He must go deep inside himself and root out the whole fabric of belief in fatigue.

He Begins to Draw Advantages

We assume our man is now free of it. He listens to his wife's story of her day—and since he is truly listening, instead of mulling around in his own problems, he hears a story or a phrase that gives him an idea for extended sales in his company. He makes a memo of it in the little book he always carries. Then he goes with his wife to a high school reception for the new principal. He isn't keen about going, but he wants to prove to himself that he can extend his sympathies away from himself.

Fine Start

At the reception or meeting, he makes a real contribution by backing up the new man's new ideas. The town profits by it— and forevermore he has the awareness that part of HIS good outgoing thinking is helping his town serve its children better, thus helping the world. Bit by bit he extends himself. Many things and people are helped and improved because of his interest. As he grows outwardly, he grows inwardly. And as he grows inwardly, he grows outwardly.

He Draws Loyalty

One day a higher-up from the home office in New York comes to town with the idea of putting a stranger above our man in the business. But the men he talks to say, "But you can't do that to Jim. He's one of the town's best-loved men. Outraged people would boycott our product." *So, even without his knowing it, his extended self has saved his family's security.*

There are so many benefits that follow self-extension. So prepare to meet your world well.

1. *Learn to speak on your feet.* (Not being able to do so ties up streams of energy.) In learning to speak well, you will pick

up phrases and new words that will be just the tools you need to put your ideas across anywhere—and you will *know* you are correct, which is always inspiring.

2. *Learn to handle your body well.*

A. Practice getting across the room to light a woman's cigarette or to greet someone. Most European men have great smoothness at this point. Their mothers have taught them, since they were little boys, to be mannerly in the presence of women. Not all American men are smooth in moving about in a room. But when they do learn to *anticipate* whatever is coming, they can be better at it than anyone. A "man of the world" sees a woman reach for a cigarette and makes *smooth moves* to give her a light, whereas the unprepared ones bang into the situation blindly, lurch upward, knocking into a vase or a chair to get there with the light. Too abrupt, too obvious.

B. Practice, actually practice, getting to your feet to bow to a woman or half-rise in a restaurant to bow to or shake hands with a man. If you are too tired to be courteous in the accepted way to women, then go home and go to bed. Don't just mull around with your shirt collar open. Do one thing or the other. Act like a gentleman or go to bed and send for a doctor. Being less than a gentleman (a superior man) simply exhausts one further.

C. Revert to your military training, and remember to stand on both feet. Lean on nothing. Men of experience, education, birth, training, position and accomplishment have a compact look, controlled, yet supple, upright without stiffness. They stand on their two feet, balanced. Nothing encourages fatigue so much as sloppy bodies, without dignity or promise or effect!

Years ago, *Life* magazine, in its center spread, published a picture of a meeting in Washington of the nation's small-business men. Several thousand men were in that picture—but from the large figures in front to the pinpoint ones in the rear of the focus, not one single man was standing on his two feet. They were all leaning on walls, tables, chairs or one another. On the next page, there was a large picture of the nation's great men in business, art, etc. The contrast was sharp. Everyone of them was standing balanced on his two feet, compact, alert, relaxed, dignified. Only one had his fists on his hips—and he was a military man, oddly enough. He looked awkward and out of place. Let's make our peace with our bodies, handle them well and forget them. But *smoothness in anything requires experience, observation and practice.*

MEN AND WOMEN WHO HANDLE THEIR BODIES WELL ALWAYS HAVE EXTRA ENERGY

There is a feeling of well-being and self-acceptance that frees energies otherwise tied up in feelings of uncertainty and awkwardness. Size has little to do with a man's grace. One of the most graceful men I have ever met was a very large man, captain of a trans-world ship. He accepted his size, danced well, and even handled a delicate glass of champagne with a controlled, simple grace (with no curled-up little finger.)

Accept your body, dress it correctly, learn to handle it gracefully, and then forget it.

Now your mind is free, energized, ready to learn about and appreciate other people. You will unavoidably be asked to take part in games. All diplomats learn the games of the countries in which they serve; also the dances and sports. One must make the effort to extend one's influence in these areas. (Homespun Benjamin Franklin won his way as a diplomat in France!)

Bridge is not necessary to one's success, but it helps. It is not greatly important at any given time that one does not play bridge. But as one gets older it becomes more important. And even young people derive a benefit from being able to accept an invitation to "make a fourth," thus, giving three other people the pleasure of a game.

There is no denying that bridge has opened many new avenues of friendships and even business and other values that broaden one's life. But, at this game, more than in any other, many people do not wish to put themselves through the embarrassments of learning. Nothing can make one feel so utterly brainless as mistakes at a bridge table that embarrass a partner.

A solution: learn quickly. To become proficient at bridge, requires much time and a long apprenticeship—a struggle that some women and many men do not wish to make. Yet, there usually comes a time when they wish they had learned it, at any cost. And for them I have a solution. One can buy a bridge-board, that is, a device by which one can play alone, privately, and untangle the mysteries and snarls of bidding and playing. You are alone (physically, that is) but at the board you are playing with three experts.

Their hands are being played through little slots in the board, so that you see how three excellent players handled the problems. You simply slide a new deal (printed on a sheet) under your board and play it through its little "windows." One can learn more bridge in two weeks with a "board" than in two years of fumbling playing with three live people. You can thus completely by-pass the awkward learning period.

Don't Say "No" When You Can Say "Yes"

I am not trying to make bridge players out of people who honestly do not like it. My aim, I am sure you know, is to remove from your life, as many negations as possible. Bridge is just a case in point. The great virtue of bridge is that you give three other people pleasure they cannot have without you.

Someone said long ago "Whenever we say 'no' we die a little." It certainly is more agreeable to be able to say "yes" as often as is consistent with our time and our desire. And I am convinced that many people say "no," pretend they don't care for it, just because they don't want to make the effort to learn, thus tying up energies that should be released. It is not true, often, that a person prefers to do something else. There is no way out of the fact that

We Enjoy Doing What We Do Well

The same thing is true of conversation, dancing, golf, riding, swimming, chess or whatever.

Standing in the receiving line at the Governor's Mansion in Raleigh, North Carolina, when Kerr Scott was Governor, I was very much amused by the advice of Daniels (son of Josephus

Daniels). "Don't give it so much, Margery," he said. "You've got to shake hands with about five thousand people. Your hand will be sore. Don't grip them. Just let them shake *your* hand. And it doesn't matter what you say. No one will know anyway. They aren't listening. They're busy with their own impressions. Just memorize a half-dozen phrases and say them one after the other.

"I proved to myself that nobody listens to what you say. I came to a reception like this years ago—and I greeted my hostess with "Good afternoon, beautiful lady. I've just done a remarkable thing. I just shot my wife." My hostess said, 'How simply fascinating. Mrs. England, may I present Mr. Daniels. He's just done something wonderful. Oh, how do you do, Mrs. Virginia.'

"I said to Mrs. England, 'I was just telling our hostess that I have just shot my wife.' She replied, 'You public figures are always doing such interesting things. Mrs. France, may I present Mr. Spaniel. His father was—Oh, how do you do, my dear.' Down the line I went through three long rooms! (Down South everybody is in the receiving line.) I told each person that I had just shot my wife. Nobody heard me. Later, I was standing in a corner alone with a cup of tea. A little woman with a puzzled expression walked up to me and said, 'Oh, Mr. Daniels, what was it you said you did? I understood you to say that you just GOT a wife. I thought you'd been married for years.' Well, we'll giver her "E" for effort. She was the only one in about a thousand who had heard anything!"

All of which may be true in a long receiving line, but in what may be even lightly termed conversation, one cannot depend on such hidden-in-plain-sight tactics. One has to have something to say.

Have Ten Remarks Ready

If one is not the chatty type, one may indeed have a few ready-made remarks that can be used pleasantly over and over. And in between, questions may be used, the answers to which will give you long time-areas in which to think of something else.

Even the most talkative people will find that the technique of drawing out others will be, in the end, the most rewarding. There is something vastly altruistic about triggering the other person's experiences and feelings in talk. You won't have to worry about his ideas—he will force them upon you!

But in the whole exchange, the basic good lies in CARING enough to be there with two eyes and two ears and to scatter as much confidence and approval as the time and your conscience allows. And you will be the "big man" or woman, the great heart, the fine adviser (though you may not have given any at all) because you provided an opportunity for the other person to think in your presence against your mind and thus clarify his thoughts himself. "They also serve, who only stand and wait."

KNOW A GOOD TOAST

However, in case you are called upon for a toast, a welcoming speech, or the defense of a point of view, you had better get ready. Why not think of it as a pleasant privilege instead of a chore? But whatever you think of it YOU ARE IT. What are you going to *do* about it? Men have built good lives on far less. Many people who think they are tired are just tired of too many blocked-off areas in their own lives. Their fatigue is far deeper than that of the one who is temporarily spent from too many errands, charities, shopping or good works. Many people need more, not less, activity in order to feel alive and strong.

There is a popular legend to the effect that entertaining is a great chore. It is about as true as that all Irishmen are red-headed. But so prevalent is the acceptance and repeated belief that hospitality is too expensive in money and energy that people bow to it like sheep caught on a fence.

Entertaining is not necessarily expensive and it isn't exhausting. But I know women and men who work themselves up to a lather before a party or (horrible words) "having company"— and afterward, rest in bed to recover! What an amazing reaction to an activity from which we would gain energy if we were not braced against it.

Preconceived Notions Are Responsible for Most Fatigue

I have always believed that when people accept an invitation to my house, dress attractively and come, bringing their most charming selves and stories, they have contributed a great amount of energy to my abode and to me. I accept it, accumulate it, value it! Why should I shut my mind to it and insist on thinking only of the amount I must spend getting ready? A big party buoys me up for a week!

There's a way to do what we want to do. During the war, living in the country, with food rationing and almost no gasoline, I learned a great deal about entertaining. Being a Southerner, I just don't feel alive if I can't have people at my board, and I learned that there are many ways of approaching the same subject. I simply refused to stop entertaining. I learned to do attractive dishes with rice and macaroni, and, of course, depended heavily on sea food. The point is that I simply flatly refused to accept the idea that we must not be hospitable.

I couldn't go along with the idea that it was extravagant, and unpatriotically hard on the nation's food supply. How silly! My guests had to eat somewhere, and they consumed no more of the nation's food at my house than they would at their own. A bit of evidence that people just don't think things through! It almost seems that some people prefer to find things difficult and moan about it.

Plan Ahead

Certainly, it stands to reason that without servants, party food must be prepared well in advance. It is better to have two or three delicious dishes than many mediocre ones. Also two or three are quite enough. If you have made your house attractive with flowers (or even arrangements of weeds, which can be very attractive and artistic) or just armfuls of green or colored leaves, a few white candles, and an open fire, your place will have charm. And if you are bright-eyed and free of culinary worries, thus focused on your guests, everyone will have a better time.

Try to plan dishes that will not be hurt by standing a bit. Be sure to have casseroles whose racks have a candle beneath to keep them warm—put them on the sideboard and don't worry!

REFRESH YOURSELF BY CHANGING YOUR CLOTHES

One thing you should insist upon: people should dress when they come to your house. It makes the evening more festive. It isn't a party if you can come in any old thing! Unless, of course, it is a picnic. Even for a swimming party, one should don attractive clothes afterward. If you value an evening at your house, other people will also gain "spirit" from it.

Don't worry about drinks. Many people think they can't entertain unless they have an array of expensive drinks including the best Scotch whiskey. I give many parties with no liquor at all. I sometimes serve champagne, but I do not consider drinks the backbone of a party. I often offer clear soup served in the living room when guests first arrive. Many of my friends give really beautiful late afternoon (on Saturday or Sunday) parties, serving only tea and sometimes coffee as drinks. The Christian Scientists never serve liquor, and many people are completely "temperance," refusing to serve any and all alcoholic beverages. Some of these people are rich and prominent. So, why not do as you please—or as your pocket-book dictates.

Tea-parties are back in vogue, and so are supper parties. After a meeting, ball or symphony, give a supper party—it's simple and easy and festive. (You're dressed anyway).

It is not necessary to exhaust yourself physically or financially to entertain. You will find that if you approach a party with joy bubbling up in your mind, you can do any amount of extra work for it without any feeling of fatigue whatever.

Thoughtless people are always saying to me "Well, aren't you just dead, after all you've done?" Of course, I am *not* just dead. I never felt better in my life. I am never happier than when people are having a good time around me. I can close my eyes and feel the happy surge of *life* all through me. Why should I be tired just because other people think I should? No thank you!

One Should Not Be Merely Gallant About Extra Efforts

That does not conquer fatigue—it merely overtaxes your physical set-up. You must be very sure that you are really revising your entire feeling about effort, from one end to the other, before you add much to your usual expenditure of energy.

I certainly do not recommend anyone's following *my* program until he has completely revised his ideas and automatic reactions to fatigue. Many people heroically add to their activities, feeling that, just to make the family happy, or for some other reason, they will agree to do many extra things. But in their hearts, they are deeply convinced that they are overdoing. And if they feel that, it is true for them.

Plan Ahead to Remove as Many Difficulties as Possible

What about your clothes? Both men and women should always keep at least one complete outfit ready at a moment's notice. It provides against the unexpected time-demand from any quarter—and relaxes a worry about not being ready. Hang the whole outfit on one hanger and with it a bag, shoes, etc. Attention in this department:

1. Frees you for other pleasures.
2. Brings you more invitations from the family (they won't have to wait).
3. Keeps the exact status of your clothes before you (no horrifying surprises).

Shakespeare was a very wise man, and one of his lines from *Hamlet* is very apropos here: "Readiness is all." *Get ready* to go, and you will have set in motion the very vibrations that will draw the rest of the matter to you.

Get ready to entertain. I usually establish a "party shelf" or cupboard. Here I keep the accessories and many of the materials I will need for an unexpected call on my hospitality. Keep quantities of paper napkins (good ones), guest towels, glasses, *et al* conveniently at hand.

It costs no more to buy canned and jarred and packaged good things leisurely in advance. You can buy them when they are "specials" and even save money by planning ahead. Buy one thing at a time. First thing you know, you will have all you need for a very good party—and it will be no particular trouble. Perhaps a certain set of silver can be polished, wrapped in black tissue paper and put away to anticipate the guests arriving in a few days.

The modern host and hostess must be prepared for unusual calls on their hospitality. One thing is certain: the more prepared one is, the less effort will be expended on meeting the challenge when it comes.

Learn to double your activities. One can read an informing book, or study a language while polishing silver, washing windows, or setting a table. One can, at any rate, put the language records on and let the teacher accustom your ears to the French idiom, or Spanish or whatever.

Impression by repetition. Speaking of languages, I have a little story to tell you. Near my washbowl is a kind of shelf, and I sometimes lay a newspaper on it to scan the headlines while I brush my teeth. For several days, once, a paper with a large tragic announcement lay there. At least a dozen times my eyes fell on this destructive headline. Suddenly, I realized that the ugly fact was being pounded into my mind by repetition. I put the thing in a waste-basket and replaced it with a French conversation book. Each time I washed my hands or face, I would glance at one phrase or another—and by gathering these otherwise lost minutes, *I advanced my study* that much.

In working on verbs, I extended the idea. I would make several copies of a declension of some verb, and, with Scotch tape, would stick them around where my eyes would naturally light on them. The multiplied impact pounded them home! One can do the same thing with lines for a play or poetry to be memorized.

USE THE REPETITIVE THEME FOR ANYTHING YOU WANT IMBEDDED IN YOUR CONSCIOUSNESS

And oppositely, see to it that tiring, discouraging, horrifying things are not repeated any oftener than can be helped. This *cleansing* of the muck and truck of contact with undisciplined people and the misfortunes of the world is a necessary part of the techniques you will have to develop if you want to keep energized. It would solve nothing for you simply to avoid the contacts. We must find the strength to meet them, but without acid criticism and without condemnation.

Society is a pleasant place. My grandmother and my mother drove this phrase home to me and made me understand that it wasn't an empty, surface thing, but a constructive foundation and attitude with which to meet life. They taught me that one has the responsibility of holding social intercourse to pleasant themes and interpretations. To burden others with our problems and heavier matters is unthinkable.

No ill nature is allowed. To quarrel in public about anything is to show one's lack of training and social experience. And we were told that it was very second rate to sit in a public place such as a restaurant and make remarks about the people who entered and left. I used to think all this was unnecessarily strict. But now I know that my people (very long-lived, by the way) had developed a way-of-going that held them to smoother, finer goals than the average; yet these goals were available to everybody. They wanted to be above the gathering of other people's mistakes or errors. To call others to task in public over real or imaginary wrongs was to show a lack of breeding. To overlook people's virtues and make much of their faults showed a mind not very sure of itself, one that must be sustained by such proppings.

Agreeableness stamps one as "desirable." It requires no money or answers to a questionnaire for anyone to join the growing numbers of men and women who have assumed the code of *pleasant people.* One finds these people everywhere. They make the world a better, more comfortable place to live in. One finds them when travelling, these jewels of serenity; *i.e.,* people who are comfortable within themselves and intend to remain that way.

GENTLE PEOPLE ATTRACT ONE ANOTHER

These people are content to let others be and do whatever suits them. They are politely willing, as someone has put it, for the leopard to have his spots and the elephant to have his trunk.

Nothing and no one from the outside can provoke or induce them to alter their course. When a member of the "club" meets another, say, in Timbuctoo, they recognize each other, and while they offer no more help to their own sort than they do to every human being they meet, they find great pleasure and strength in the meeting.

Gentle people do seem to gravitate together, as water flows downhill. They can sense the presence of someone else who is angled toward harmony and gentleness. Mind you, they don't expect perfection. They ask only which way your attention and desire is turned: toward the selfish, sensual, and destructive, or toward that which is basically harmonious and gentle and therefore strong and dependable.

MOST OF LIFE'S BENEFITS THAT HAVE REACHED ME HAVE COME TO ME BECAUSE OF MY DEDICATION TO THAT SIDE OF THE PICTURE

In a world that may, at any moment, burst into the flames of war, one must do some deep soul-searching to determine the way one shall go through an experience of violence, treachery, and false representations. The need is all the greater for controls and self-management, lest we retrograde too deeply into the animal and jungle strata of awareness.

In peace or war, we must daily, every hour, every minute, make the choice between the fine and the coarse, and *only* as we take the higher path in the tiny ways open to us, can we train our sensibilities toward the greater issues.

Most people are basically noble. Why do we want more energy? Is it not that we truly want to do more for others—our families, our communities, our world? The very fact that we want more strength in order to GIVE more would get it for us if we did not concentrate on our emptiness and lack instead of our great potential.

Selflessness and generosity as evidenced in entertaining shows the yearning of the human heart to express largeness through giving. And it becomes ever easier once we have gone beyond the struggle with the idea that it is difficult.

Cultivate an atmosphere of festivity. A fete day is one in which some fine idea is celebrated. Some cynic once said that the fact that we have fete days shows how far we are from any high-mindedness the rest of the time. At any rate, the remark does remind us that we should not wait for Sunday to celebrate the love of our God. We should not wait for a date in May to appreciate our mothers, or, in June, our fathers. And Easter? Why have it only once a year? Every time the Christ within (our consciousness of Sonship) is lifted above the discord of earth, it is the victory of Easter. It should happen many times a day!

These days are all very fine—and far better than nothing. But what about tuning our minds to heroism, to selflessness, to the service of others, to concentration on beauty and all the other lovely thoughts that are ours for the taking EVERY DAY? *Joy is the feeling that sends our blood surging through our veins, bringing LIFE and carrying off waste.*

Why not make a great occasion of every day, every meal? Why not look as well as possible and move and speak acceptably at every meal? Why not have the habit of happiness? Someone has said that even dying is just a bad habit! Why not make a deliberate effort to cultivate fine habits, especially in sharing with others?

At a party, one wouldn't dream of focusing on anyone's faults; one would, by appreciation and drawing out the best of each guest, inspire him to find splendid things within himself. This is the real purpose of having guests. So why not practice for it? Have several rehearsals at your own table. Why not perfect the idea?

Have a family party tonight. Have a favorite dish of each member of the family, if possible. Spruce up just a little. The boys and father will wear their coats. And they will seat mother and the girls—even though mother may have to get up to attend to the rest of the dinner (though she could arrange that to a minimum with a little planning.)

The major objectives are:

1. Appreciate the food without gobbling it.

2. Speak only of pleasant matters; no one's faults are to be aired. No one is to be scolded, just this once, not even with firm looks.

3. Work each person's virtues into the conversation somehow.

4. If you have no immediate pleasantries to discuss, speak of those of other people. Reminisce or project something wonderful ahead.

5. Put all sensitiveness aside. Do not imagine that other people's virtues are discussed to make you feel inferior. You have your own virtues.

6. For this one hour, do not think of yourself at all; devote it to making others happy.

I promise you that all will not go smoothly this first time. Someone will be bored. Someone will be unable to keep his mind off himself, or will find offense at something. Someone may leave the room in tears because in some way he feels he is not measuring up and is conspicuous for it. All sorts of things can go wrong until the whole family catches the spirit of "entertaining" one another.

These rehearsals can well be the prelude to a successful life. Not because one expects to go to parties endlessly, but because the disciplines are far more demanding than they may at first appear. But the great benefit is the training of the mind to respond to, and to look for, the worthy, the pleasant, the agreeable—a practice that will lift any life to new heights, raise the prestige of a family, and in the end bring honor and distinction.

Certainly there will be the usual number of catcalls. But if a man stopped training himself just because of the voices on the sidelines he would never get to first base. Think of the catcalls any prominent person must endure. But he also, in due time, receives honors, appointments, responsibilities—and has many inner satisfactions, to say nothing of the material rewards. Also, he is training himself to think away from himself, clearing his mind for any issues he must consider as a man in an important position.

The Quality of Survival

The attitudes I have been describing in this chapter were the code of my family and relatives. As I have already told you, they were very long-lived people. Oddly enough, there were no divorces among them, not because they "didn't believe in divorce" but because they made their marriages happy ones. I invited some cousins from down South to visit me in New York a few years ago. They declined, saying, "We are now in our eighties, but our calendar is so full that we cannot get to New York this year. Perhaps we could come next year if you ask us again. We are both free of the disabilities that commonly go with age and are active in many ways."

"The quality of survival is suffused with positive qualities and has little to do with negations." This was a remark of my father's. How dramatically its truth has been brought home to us during the wars of our lifetime! People who had had training in pleasant thinking and living politely survived the most grilling tests far more often than those who had not that inner discipline and richness.

A Giant's Strength

So these are not "cream puff attitudes" or just something for rich people or those fortunately placed. There is a giant's strength in the man who can put off discord, who really believes that people are good underneath and that God's world is a dependable, orderly and receptive place. This man can endure, sometimes for years, being shut up in a prison or otherwise confined. He devotes himself to the welfare of others and saves his own soul, mind, and often his body.

I have met some survivors from refugee camps. Those who

had disciplined minds to start with seemed to be able to find a well-spring of energy and faith. They were able to keep their children informed of their heritage in this way. In the long, dull evenings they taught their children to memorize poetry! Not only did the memorizing fill their minds with pleasurable thoughts to lighten the empty sadness of their position, but the exercise it provided kept their minds bright and keen. It put off the deterioration that is commonly supposed to be the lot of a prisoner after a number of years.

Pleasant things in the mind enable one to entertain others and to be entertained oneself.

SUPPOSE YOU WERE GOING TO BE CAST AWAY ON A DESERT ISLAND, WITH YOUR WIFE AND CHILDREN

If there were an atomic attack and you had to live confined in a very limited space, how would *you* fare? Do you have material enough stored away in your head to educate, train, preserve and elevate others and yourself? It is a choice one makes. Create within yourself a storehouse of delights and values. May you never need them in a prison or atomic camp! But those same values will give you their strength and support in a long life. The years will be such good ones that you will not find them tiring.

GET READY with inner riches that will keep you sane in difficulties, enhance your value as a citizen of the world, and make you a giant among men.

Strange, isn't it, that the same clean gathering of the strength of beauty that will enhance you as a public figure will stand by you in a prison or under limited conditions. There must be a kinship here with the basic creative Mind of the universe. It must be a small ray from the mind of God that lights these attitudes and practices of living.

10

WHAT IS YOUR MT. EVEREST?
CLIMB IT!

Who with his might aspires unto the mountain's upper height
Holds in that aspiration a great trust to be fulfilled.

Emilie Cady

Deep in almost every heart is one highest, keenest, unfulfilled desire. The amount of pressured energy backed up behind that desire is enough for two careers. If you are extremely tired, it could well be because most of your energy is syphoned off into the plugged channel of this frustrating hope, urge, or desire.

To wait, wait, wait for the fruition of some dream often becomes, in time, a drama of disappointment, emptying, drying, dulling, exhausting. It has been an inextinguishable flame that burned only a part of the energy it drew around itself. Fortunately, there are many determined people who never surrender their dream to despair and despondency. Faith and tenacity are the qualities needed.

There is always a way to arrive at some version of your goal. It is never too late—well, almost never. Since everything begins with an idea, a mental pattern, it is plain that ideas were meant by nature to reach fulfillment, objectification. If your cherished plan has remained unrealized, it may be because you have not been doing very much about it. Or it may be that the mountain looked too high and too risky to attempt.

Your deep desire may, at the beginning, have been a creation of the sum of your latent talents. It could have been colored by your education. It could have been inspired by someone,

105

a lecturer, an actor, a neighbor, a great world figure, whom you saw but once, or perhaps not at all. But a flame was lighted in your mind—a flame that, for a time, leaped and burned with bright, clear design. The years passed. The flame became coals —and at night, when you cannot sleep, you sometimes stir the coals, and once again your old ideal flows across the screen of your mind and looms large.

A happy experience or self-torture. For some people this "dream revisited" is a happy experience, but for others it can be a time of self-blame and torture, or of blaming others for the fact that the dream is still unrealized. For too many, the light of hope slowly goes out, taking their strength with it. These weary-with-waiting ones are so tired—so deeply tired! These are the tragic ones!

The ones who enjoy dreaming their dream never give up their pleasure in thinking about it. And whether or not they know it, they are moving slowly toward it. For them it has a sense of reality. They accept its feasibility somehow.

Events move toward and into a stubbornly held dream. For every person who can tell a story of ill luck that made his goal impossible—accidents, obligations and illnesses that moved it beyond his reach—there are thousands who kept right on climbing, and eventually reached the top of their own Mt. Everest.

The spirit of the times is to rise above all handicaps. We have doctors in wheelchairs, who are socially popular as well. Dr. Clifford Wright of Los Angeles has a large practice in internal medicine, is active in civic groups, and is seen at many parties and balls. He is witty, gracious, very much sought after as a dinner guest. He was a victim of polio many years ago. After a very grim inner battle, he decided to go right ahead and to live life to its fullest. He married a charming widow with two children. Their family life is delightful and valuable to the community and nourishing to their many admiring friends. He is a man who would not take "no" for an answer.

We have research scientists who are without legs. We have blind people in all manner of valuable work, from psychiatry to musical and dramatic criticism! We know now as we have never known before that LIFE is determined in the mind.

Time is unimportant. Events may slow down your progress, but if you keep on moving in the right direction, your pace is not too important. I know a young man who was studying law at New York University when his supporting uncle died. Instead of leaving college, as many less-determined men usually do under such circumstances, he took a dish-washing job at night to pay for his food. And so it goes! Another young man learned to play the trumpet and literally blew his way through an education in medicine.

It may be easier to settle for another kind of job, marry the girl, put a down payment on a house and go on from there. But the growing spirit awakened in the land is the one of challenge and service. Oldsters and youngsters are stirred anew by the soul-searching question, "How can I make my life count for the most for the world?"

THE NEW CHALLENGES ARE BASED ON THE HIGHEST COMMON DENOMINATOR, NOT THE LOWEST

Too much security gets to be a great bore, they say. Anyway, what is security, and who really has it? These questions are replacing the rat races of the faint-hearted.

The best advice for a young man is to pick out a girl who also has a dream, marry her, and together, with supporting confidence and affection, climb your Everest hand in hand. Shun the ones who are looking for a soft place. Look for the old pioneer spirit, which is far from dead in both sexes. (Two of my great-grandmothers helped fire at attacking Indians from behind lace curtains, dressed in ball-gowns.) I suggest that all young men read Stephen Vincent Benét's description of a Southern "lady" in his epic poem "John Brown's Body." Two simple, but priceless, lines from it are: "She knew her Bible, and how to flirt" and "to manage a gentleman's whole plantation/in a manner befitting her female station." These are but tidbits from the banquet of the book.

Everyone's timing is different. Everyone must make his peace with the time element in his own life. It may be like no one else's, but if we do not sink under comparing ourselves with swifter, more "fortunate" colleagues, we can reach our goal too. We are too likely to expect our efforts to bring us out into victory before they have had a real chance to mature into skill and accomplishment. We are too impatient with life—too impatient with ourselves.

We plant the seeds, but it is not we who make them grow. We must wait for the natural processes to complete their inherent cycles of development. When we let ourselves despair, we truly lose touch with these natural forces, and they—and we—die slowly. This giving up, this denial of the saving factors in life, is a real and definite blasphemy, as we have said. It is an insulting commentary on God's created world. It is a condemnation of the laws of the universe.

No curse could be more absolute than to lose all faith in the processes of life. As we lose faith, we lose energy—and as we lose energy, we lose faith. How sad to be so blind! A little more patient faith and many a life would find its balance again.

When anyone "gives up," it is always too soon. There is scarcely a hotel man in the world who cannot tell you several experiences in his hostelry that bear out this truth. More than once, some anxious guest, whose strained hopes are focused on the outcome of a single deal or situation, has one day despaired of a solution—and has taken his life. Perhaps minutes or hours later, a telegram of acceptance or letter of hope and help has been pushed under his door. When the authorities have broken into the room, they have found the body and the saving telegram lying, sometimes, only inches apart. No words can add to the effect of that tableau.

But whether the saving message lies right at hand, or not, LIFE offers itself to every man, with its responsive, ever-giving, dependable laws of creativity!

THERE IS ALWAYS A WAY THAT NATURE'S LAWS
CAN BRING A SATISFACTORY SOLUTION

There is a way out of every dilemma. Whatever the immediate wreckage or tragedy, LIFE flows on, with its unrealized, unknown forces unused by man.

As the sun rises and the seasons roll, LIFE pushes into expression, no matter what limitations man's opinion tries to superimpose upon it. The drama of diminishment and failure is in *him,* not in life's processes.

Write another act to your personal drama when tragedy threatens you, in which you turn to the changing, flowing forces available to you, and shape them to your desire—this time having humility enough to work WITH natural law, and not against it. The tragedy, whatever it is, may never come; but even if it did, it would be only an *experience,* while you, *the experiencer,* shall live to create a finer epilogue.

Values are inherent in everything. In "Gone With The Wind," one of Rhett Butler's most cynical lines bore a great truth. I have forgotten the exact words, but the gist of them was that there was as much profit to be made while a nation was being wrecked as when it was expanding. In other words nothing in the world is valueless.

Success can, and often does, rise like the phoenix from ashes. There is no failure and no loss in nature. There is only the continual process of making something new. Why not use this law instead of letting it break you when the real tests come?

This is in no sense a pep-talk. It is a statement of the wonderful world in which we live and which we can shape, if we will find the faith to lay hold of it and command it. The very fact that you have a concept of some fine goal indicates that you are potentially capable of it. But, be willing to travel the road to it! Be willing to work in faith and wait for the processes of growth toward it. "Wait!" you may say. "I've been doing that most of my life. I'm tired of waiting." You must learn to wait expectantly and dynamically, not dismally.

What was your dream? What is your dream? Start toward it again, if you want to overcome fatigue. I know a man who was a semi-invalid. He had always wanted to travel to the so-called cradles of civilization, the Euphrates valley, India, Egypt, Persia, the Greek islands, to learn of the past. But every time he saved some money for the trip, a family crisis would come along and absorb all of it. He started over and over again—

and got nowhere. Gradually, his whole personality began to sag.

This man came to me for interviews, ostensibly to gain social ease, but actually (in his words) to "break the jinx" of his habitual frustrations. He was not a stupid man. He *knew* the law of mental causation. He could see it operating in other people's lives. He had not so clear a view of his own situation.

He said to me, "You claim that a mental picture carried over a certain period of time will find its way into one's experience. In theory, I agree, but look at me! I've thought about travel to far places and being an archeologist most of my life—and that's as far as I get."

HOW SUBTLE ARE THE LAWS OF MIND! HOW EXACT!

Under careful and slow questioning, it became apparent that this man had never really *believed* he would get there. Here is his real story.

Buried deep in his mind was a neurotic fear of the desert. He was afraid of sand, because when he was a little boy of five he had dug a passage in a dune near his family's beach place, and it had caved in on him. He was terrified of holes, and possible landslides. He wanted to know what was buried in these ancient lands, but his revulsion to the process of finding out by digging had negated his mental pattern. We did not discover this at once, but it gradually became clear. We both believed that we had found the root of his problem.

However, a basic, hidden revulsion can have many involved and tangled outgrowths, each of which is like a tiny thread of no particular strength, but all of which combined are able to trip up a man and change the direction of his life.

For instance, this man's wife and his mother were enthusiastic gardeners. They preferred to do their planting in the late afternoon, when he was at home from work. They always called on him to help. So basically distasteful was the very act of shovelling loose dirt that he would invent headaches—and once even broke an ankle—to avoid it.

He was not consciously aware of what he was doing to himself. The more he suffered from his dislike of a shovel and dirt, the stronger grew the dislike, and the firmer became the determination to avoid it!

His accumulating dislike finally extended to the flowers and vegetables that were to be planted. One by one, he stopped eating vegetables. He began to collect allergies to flowers. On and on his tangles went. His diet of meats and sweets soon had his digestive tract troubled, which encouraged the allergies. A number of "vicious circles" were established. The involvements were incredible!

How could his hope of being an archeologist become a reality with all those crossed wires? Patiently training his mind to dislike nothing, eating first one vegetable and then another, thereby showing himself that they were really delicious, he gradually broke down the network of revulsion.

He grew up emotionally, and put away the childishness of his fear. "When I became a man, I put away childish things." (1st Corinthians 13-11.) Facts dispel illusion. Understanding relaxes fear and causes it to disappear as a mist before the sun.

TO BE REALLY GROWN-UP IS TO BRUSH ALL DISLIKES ASIDE, FOR DISLIKE IS ANOTHER NAME FOR FEAR; IT WEARS A THOUSAND FACES

No man can climb his particular Mt. Everest, that defying peak of high desire, if he harbors fear. All your reasons why you think you cannot reach your goal are but rationalized fears. GROW UP, start on your climb of self-mastery, and slowly reach your great possibility.

Merely shifting dislikes is not conquering them. An interesting side-effect of the dislikes of the man we were discussing was this mental twist: when he saw the wisdom of conquering his dislike of vegetables and flowers, the first (and very much to be expected) move was merely to shift his mass of dislikes from one point to another. In this case, the shift was from flora to fauna (from plant to animal life). The pivotal fact here is that an emotion will always find some object or victim on which to rest. The only permanent cure is to get rid of the emotion itself.

Our man, when he decided against disliking vegetables and flowers, simply moved his habit-demand of revulsion over to the human beings in his life. He began to find fault with his wife. First one thing about her and then another he found wrong. She couldn't please him. His children's noise became unbearable to him. His mother-in-law was put out of the house —but that wasn't too important.

One can always find something "unbearable" when that demand becomes an automatic necessity. First one employee and then another left in tears. Finally, his wife went to a lawyer to see about a divorce. I stopped that. But before I could convince him that he must uproot the feeling of distaste he was developing for everybody who came near him, he had made some unfortunate moves in antagonizing business people. What a time he had to retrieve the advantages he himself had torn apart!

He finally won back his business gains, his family harmony, and victory over his own emotions. He really had the intelligence, maturity and humility to see that the entire drama was being played INSIDE himself. And INSIDE himself the corrections must be made. He was man enough to do it, I am happy to relate.

Today, he is a happy, successful, distinguished archeologist. I wish I could give you his name, but I have not his permission. He is perfectly healthy. For relaxation, he works in his garden, wherever he finds himself. Wherever he goes he plants one! He has no allergies now.

This same success is open to anyone who is willing to be honest with himself and to work at correcting his errors. Being honest with oneself is the hardest part. Of course, there is that occasional person who goes to extremes in condemning himself. He tries to mix sympathy-getting hopelessness with his "honesty." He is likely to say, in a kind of blanket coverage, trying to baffle accusations from within and without, "I'm just as wrong as I can be. It's my nature. I've always been wrong. I'll always BE wrong—and what can you do about it?" One's impulse is to say, "Oh, grow up!" Instead, one must take him seriously and try to help.

Every "jinx" is a do-it-yourself job. The "jinx" our man thought he had was simply a network of his own reactions. One has to work hard to cut across the beneficent laws of salutary response active in us and in our world!

WE ARE DEALING WITH LAW AT EVERY POINT IN LIFE— KINDLY LAW, IT SEEMS, BUT LAW

It is the child in one that wants to ignore the established process, to kick over the traces, and have what he wants when he wants it. One of the saddest sights in the world is a talented, clever person trying to make his own laws—and trying to make them fit his weaknesses, not his strengths. Though he may squirm this way and that, the values of his abilities leak away from him. He becomes bruised by his failures and pretends (he may even have convinced himself) that the goal doesn't interest him! By working *with* the law of any process, we can make it serve our ends.

Whatever you now have is the result of the working of the law of cause and effect. If you are tired, you are doing the things, thinking the thoughts, feeling the emotions that keep you exhausted. What you feel is the definite result of definite causation.

WHY NOT SET IN MOTION THE LAWS THAT WILL FULFILL YOUR HOPES; WHY GIVE THEM UP

As you have observed, all the dams and destroyers of fulfill-ment are rooted in fear, doubt, selfishness or despair. These are more deadly than the Four Horsemen of the Apocalypse. And the blackest of these eating "sins" is *despair*. We have already called it blasphemy. But, for those who don't mind a little blasphemy, let us speak of it in terms of its chemistry, as it withers whatever it touches.

Despair is on the list of cardinal sins in the annals of the Catholic Church. It belongs on every list of attitudes to avoid as one would try to escape a highly dangerous disease. It is a self-determined emptiness. It is turning the back on all hope of rescue. It is the irreducible minimum of the human concept.

How dare you despair! By what right do you condemn a truly beneficent and helping, giving world? No matter how rampant are the evils brought upon us by barbaric, selfish, animalistic men, the stream of constructive healing and "becoming" flows on, and on, and on.

Not everyone's Mt. Everest is a world-shaking career. For many men, it is the conquering of a destructive habit, a bad temper, or a narcotic. Excesses and extremes must be shaped into line, too. Some people wish to dis-enslave themselves from cigarettes, overeating or just laziness.

NOTHING ON EARTH CAN WITHSTAND THE WILL OF MAN, HIS DEFINITE DECISION

If he makes up his mind to a certain end, and faithfully performs the demands of its laws, he will dominate the matter, sooner or later. Oddly enough, when he becomes master of himself, the outer challenges loom not so large, so terrifying or discouraging.

To a man who conquers himself, Mt. Everest looks much easier to climb.

When one has proved to himself that he is truly running himself, and not being run by habits, fears, expediency or compulsions, his mind reaches out to discover his world, his universe. Energy instantly flows in and around his extended grasp.

Energy is enthusiasm, curiosity, the thrill of the game. If you want to know what lies over the horizon (within or without) take a notch in your belt, whistle a tune, and go find out! Your horizon may be on an Eastern ocean, an expanding business, a painting, or the secrets of a test-tube. It is wherever you have put it. But it is *your* horizon.

Measure your strengths when you are preparing to start. I

they are good enough, don't delay. If they aren't, wait until you have brought them up to par for the trip. It is your strengths that will take you over the top. So, concentrate on them, instead of on your weaknesses. Thinking overmuch of your faults will bring you finally to a feeling of inadequacy. They will blind your eyes to your possibilities and quash your courage.

I know it is supposed to be modest and becoming to be keenly aware of your lacks; but if you live with them constantly, you'll die. Think wisely, instead, of your capacities. And build up, in whatever way is needed, your strengths. Which way are you looking: toward your faults, or toward your possibilities? Keep these thoughts very much to yourself. Supply whatever you need, and stop worrying.

Forget the reasons why not—and make a list of the reasons why you can! You'll never hit a target with your back turned to it. If there is a marsh of lack between you and the shore you want to reach, then build a bridge!

Do you need more knowledge of a subject? Do you need a college degree? Go back and get it! Any number of people of all ages have gone back to school. You may feel self-conscious, but after the first day, no one will pay any attention to you. They are too busy with their own problems.

Trying to meet life without proper preparation is exhausting. Do not take "no" for an answer from life at any point. If you can't make one plan work, then find a more yielding way. My nurse down South used to say to me, "Honey, there is moah ways of killin' a cat than chokin' it on butter."

If someone expresses the opinion that your way of solving your problem looks peculiar, just stare him down! A wager could be laid that his inner problems are more of a problem to him than yours are to you. Just go on your way stubbornly and serenely. Time will pass—it's a habit it has—and one day you will be sitting atop your Mt. Everest.

Take your time. Think about it. Plan. Draw it out. Write it out. Make endless lists and projections. Expenses? What can you use instead of money? Go as slowly as you must, but go. Prepare yourself for your dream.

THE WORDS "TOO LATE" DO NOT EXIST FOR THE PERSON WHO TRULY UNDERSTANDS THE WAY THE UNIVERSE WORKS

At any time, a firm decision and clear picture become the nucleus which will draw to itself new energies, new materials and new participants—or cause the old ones to return full of new life. The response is NEW, in any case.

Put yourself on the right road—and then trust it. Though you may not be able to see encouraging signposts at any given time that tell you how far you have gone, just doggedly put one foot in front of the other steadily, knowing that even a snail would cover the ground eventually.

Time works with us when we stop dreading it. It's earlier than you think! Draw deep down into your bodily and mental lungs the strong currents of the atmosphere you want there. Do not listen to the carping voices of the discouragers. They're always around. It's a way they have of compensating for their failures.

Almost all cynicism, almost all low concepts of life or people are really groans of pain. People who indulge in them are really saying "ouch." Do not permit them to influence your decision, your speed or your objective. Go your own inwardly sure way! But do not believe that it will always be smooth. The way will become rough at times.

There will be people, like Job's wife and some of his friends, who will point out the difference, the disparity, between your dedication and your present advance. You will recall that Job's wife finally cried out to him as he lay in a gutter, covered with sores, "Curse God and die!" Perhaps these very words were needed to reveal to Job that that was exactly what he was doing. He immediately took the opposite stand and rose to his magnificent "I KNOW that my redeemer liveth." And again, "Though He slay me, yet will I trust Him."

Job's stubborn, passionate faith in the basic goodness of God and His universe brought about the only possible result of its strong purity. He met every loss, every temptation, every indignity with inwardly held belief in ultimate good, complete faith in the processes of life.

SUCH CLEAR ARTICULATION OF THE PRINCIPLE OF LIFE
ALWAYS BRINGS THE SAME RESULT

The story is the same, whether you give good and evil the names of persons or the names of elements and techniques. The mechanics of the way faith draws upon universal ENERGY operate no matter what names are used. In Job, the story of this struggle is a fine dramatization, one of the best pieces of literature in the world.

Take a fresh look at your own Mt. Everest and say, "HM! doesn't look so high!" The moment you say this sincerely, you will have begun to release all the pent-up energy that was held back by doubt, indifference and despair. Ideas, ways and means will turn in your mind and sparkle in the light of new acceptance.

Did you want a house in the country? Did you want to master music? Did you dream of being an actor, a scientist, a missionary, a minister, a doctor, a writer, a painter? Did you want businesses or travel and study abroad? Did you try often, and come to the conclusion that it was not for you? Try again— and this time, with fresh impetus, vast patience, and gentle, but granite stubbornness.

Persistence is your best ally. Sometimes one thinks, "Well, it didn't work before, why should it succeed now?" There are any number of reasons. I have seen a stonemason strike a rock, trying to break it, fifteen or twenty times; then draw back to study the stone, for perhaps ten minutes. Then, carefully, he would pick up his mallet and give a very casual blow on the spot he had decided was the key point—and lo, the stone fell apart in two equal halves.

You have been learning many things in the years since you let your dream gather dust. You have much more experience, richness, and control to bring to it now. Perhaps you now know just the point to strike! Or you *could* know it if you would put doubt, self-depreciation and your ideas of ill luck or fate aside. Why not believe in your successful destiny? Do not accept any other.

Most great world figures succeeded just as long as they be-

lieved in their good luck and high destiny. The moment they began to listen to soothsayers who planted doubt in their minds, they lost their magic grip on the moving forces that respond *exactly* to ideas. This was true of Caesar. His belief in his destiny was all-encompassing. Recall the story of the fearful sailor in whose boat he was crossing a body of water in a storm? Caesar laughed loudly. "What have you to fear? You carry Caesar!" They landed safely. Who knows but that seepings of doubt of his continuing "luck" kept him from listening to the warnings about the Ides of March, and made him vulnerable? One wonders if even treachery could have reached him, if no cracks had appeared in his inner armor of belief in himself. Indeed, food for thought.

It is said that Napoleon believed in "luck." Stories persist that Hitler, Mussolini and Peron consulted soothsayers frequently. Superstition could have weakened the magnificent hold on self-confidence all these men once had. Under its power-stealing sway, logic was diluted and tactical errors made. Noise and bravado do not necessarily indicate full belief in oneself. One can go on yelling one's taunts and challenges without outward show of doubt, yet inwardly there may be a slackening of one's grip on full faith in the outcome. Some men cannot be "reasoned" into failure. Others (more) cannot be reasoned into success. The latter remind us of the woman who said to her husband, "Now, don't confuse me with facts. I've made up my mind!"

LESSON FROM A CIRCUS MAN

P. T. Barnum, circus man and impresario extraordinary, saw all he possessed burned to the ground thirteen times before he really made his fortune. But when he died, a large portion of the city of Bridgeport, Connecticut bore his mark. Today, there are hotels there, boulevards, city blocks, parks and other places that bear his name.

How could any man keep up his courage and his faith when ill luck so dogged his footsteps that he lost everything thirteen times—and yet have the mental energy to try again! I'm sure that most of us would not go on after the third or fourth burning out. But here was a man who had a dogged belief that someday, somehow, he would strike just the right combination of talents, weather, and population and all would be splendid. He refused to believe in ill luck. He kept hammering at the stone of success until he cleaved it in two. He believed in people. He believed in his business. He believed in himself. And, so far as anyone knows, he never wavered.

LESS TIME TO DOUBT IN THE JET AGE—
AND THE SWIFTER WORLD TO COME

The wisdom of stripping the inner emotions of as much conflict as possible is patent in a world that makes more and more demands on us. Survival demands as little deadwood as we can manage. Split-second decisions will be necessary to dispose of the question in hand, for others are arising before us in a matter of minutes. Not only must our load be light for the long haul, but it must be minimal because of the speed we must have. Only a clean, light, well-trained, well-oriented mind can keep its balance, make accurate decisions, synchronize its movements with thousands of others in split seconds. This and more will be the MUST of the man of the future—and not such a distant future.

We must have done with fatigue, that great planter of doubts. When we feel strong we can throw off the world's constant suggestion of diminishment and defeat. We can throw off our own tendency to take that tone. But when we collect the clutter and corrosion of disappointment, hurt, unrequited love and unsatisfied, infantile ego-hungers, we weaken our faith in our efforts and lives. We build up a fatigue that is an invitation to disaster.

If you would be strong, build up a dogged faith in yourself, your inner self. Do not be argued into listlessness by a calendar or a clock or anybody's idea of when or how things should happen, how long it should take, or who gets the credit. DO NOT ACCEPT YOUR FORMER DEFEAT-ESTIMATE OF YOUR POWERS.

Form a program that will train your mind to vigorous re-

sponse to your calls upon it. Do not imagine that a passing agreement with these truths will avail much. They have to be drilled into your unconscious reflexes. There is work to be done to uproot old habits, old sensitivities and old responses. It is a good practice to assert your position in silent thought often during the day, and before retiring at night. Only by repeated claim can a definite channel be made in your thought patterns to hold the flow of ideas where you want them.

You want support and strength when you need it in your climb. You want good habits to back you up when you are under a strain. Never let your mind waver this way and that, picking up suggestions, emotions, attitudes that do not further your hopes and plans. Your mental strength must be so vivid and vital that it can survive the onslaught of a few unavoidable disappointments.

Since the tendency of the human mind is to be influenced by passing, flimsy evidence, strength of purpose must be developed, just as muscular habits that are good should be developed in the body. The mind, being man's most precious possession, should definitely be conditioned to salutary conclusions. Mental health demands the establishment of thought habits that are in the last as well as the first analysis, GOOD.

Raise your sights. Focus on your particular Mt. Everest. There are three major conclusions necessary to put you in line with your trip up that grade. They are:

1. That it is *your* trip, even though many have made it before.

2. That you have been by-passing it long enough.

3. That you, and only you, can make that special trip, because it is a part of you.

Once these are settled firmly, you will gather the tools and equipment, choose the maps, talk to men who know about it, and decide, completely absorbed, on all the details that will guarantee you a safe, sure and successful trip.

THIS THING YOU REALLY WANT TO DO

You will be embarking on the most peculiarly personal appointment of your life. It is your responsibility to do what you were born to do. Improve your talents. Accomplish something of value to yourself, your family and/or the world. You didn't come here to shirk it. You didn't come here to be a beachcomber. You came here to use the wonderful brain you were given. You came here to carve order and harmony out of what will remain chaos if you renege. You came to take another step in man's upward climb from savagery to soul and complete mastery. Your own goal is simply the way you will go to do it.

Remember the parable of the buried talent. But that story does not even hint at the suffering a man can pull down on himself by procrastination, by rationalizing and shifting blame. Why not take command of the whole thing and start toward that mountain peak? It means self-mastery, skills, arts, works, hazards and joys, setbacks and spurts until your Mt. Everest is reached.

Shake off all foggy sense of fatigue as though it were the dust of years. Emerge from it sentient, clean, ready. No one is going to talk you out of it this time! Your decision has drawn and released floods of energy, eternal strength, the might of the movement of *mind*. If you want to rest, you'll rest. But you will proceed knowing that you are gathering force as well as spending it.

You're through with the burden of being tired. You're happier than you have ever been, because you're free of excuses, delays. You are your own man!

STAY ON THE ROAD. DON'T LOSE YOUR WAY.
BON VOYAGE!

11

TURNING THE YEARS BACK

HOW TO HOLD OR RETAIN THE FRESHNESS OF YOUTH

Vigor, endurance, tirelessness: these are the attractive features of youth to those who may have found them waning. Not everyone wants to look like a college boy or girl, but we would certainly like to keep in excellent repair, to look fresh and to feel strong.

NATURE'S GREAT PREOCCUPATION IS CREATIVITY

As we have already noted, nature seems interested only in the new creation. In animate and inanimate objects she appears almost to want to seek disintegration, since there is a tendency for all established things to slide into "ruins" unless they are very well tended. We must learn to deal with this tendency.

NATURE'S MOVEMENT IS FORWARD

Again, as already noted, nature has spread before us the few, but very strict, rules by which we can put off the disintegrating process in ourselves. We must put ourselves where nature's forward-moving forces and laws can operate to our advantage.

WE MAY NOT OPPOSE THE WAY NATURE WORKS

We have seen that a clean cell which is also well fed, can endure limitlessly. We have seen that we must obey the physical laws of that cell—but we must also attend to the emotions and ideas that color its ambience.

MOVE!

A "young" muscle is resilient, because it has been fed that which it needed, and has had sufficient movement to keep it pliant and to agitate its debris out of it. What do we learn from this? Exactly—*move!* Probably the most difficult lesson our children learn is to keep still! Somewhere along the line we overdo it and become dangerously *inactive*. Watch children.

They skip down the street. Why don't you wait until after dark and skip with them? Oh, you're afraid of what our other inactive, stodgy friends would think of you. Of course, one can get a skipping rope and use it on the back porch, but just how does one go about accompanying that with the feeling of joyousness the children obviously feel when they skip? I'm afraid one without the other might get the same fractional result. So do the next best thing and turn on some music and skip to a lovely rhythm.

Take a long, loving look at that skipping rope. It is such a good friend of man—far and away above the dog. (Unless you let your dog take you for good runs—not walks.) That little rope—it still can be bought for a dime—will save you a fortune. Have you any idea how much a good liver stirrer-upper costs when you buy it from a reliable druggist with a fancy doctor's prescription? A miracle drug, the fruit of some scientist's patient research, naturally has to be paid for. But (now don't laugh) your ten-cent rope will do almost the same thing, as nature meant it to be done, mechanically, instead of chemically.

But, of course, you must start in time. Don't wait until you have a disturbance from too much inaction, rich food, alcohol and gradual dissipation. The inaction is probably the worst of the lot—and next would be the food.

TAKE RESPONSIBILITY FOR YOUR STATE OF HEALTH AND TAKE IT NOW

Give your body:
1. Movement. And see that you enjoy it.
2. Liquids. Go on a liquid diet one day a week.

3. Fresh fruits and vegetables. Take all you can tolerate.
4. Plenty of proteins—not all from meat.
5. "Friendly bacteria" from buttermilk, yogurt and such cultures to offset the unfriendly bacteria you unconsciously get.
6. Oxygen. Straighten up and breathe deeply.
7. Bright expectations. Drop worry and focus on a fine future.

There are many ramifications and interpretations under these seven headings. But these are the magic formula for health and youth. Any definite deviation from this supply of necessities will cost you much, too much, in the end. These are "iron demands." You may get most of your "movement" while sitting almost still with the exercises I have given you, or you may get out in track pants in the early morning and jog a mile or so, but you MUST DO SOMETHING or else!

Water! Water!

I have acquaintances who drink little or no water, and all of them have expensive ailments (dehydrated people are not long-lived). Yet, they brag about how little water they drink! I don't understand it! Apparently, the human mind will boil up pride in anything unusual which it hopes is outstanding.

Since the body itself is about eighty per cent liquid, it stands to reason that one had better respect its great demand for moisture. I often tell students, "Whenever you think of me, mentally see me offering you a glass of water."

On rising, go to the tap and drink a glass of water, hot or cold, whichever you like best. After you are dressed, take another. And as soon as you arrive at the office or wherever you go, have another. In between, you will have had coffee or tea with your breakfast, plus some fruit juice. Now you are ready for your day.

Stay Young! Keep Fresh! Energy Follows!

In many ways getting old is a process of "drying up." It certainly looks that way. Naturally it is an action of complicated causes, but why not dilute them, whatever they are! By watering down any poisons you may have in your system, you give your body a chance to handle them and it will probably win against them, especially if you supply the other six items in the formula.

There's nothing very new about this formula. The refreshing point here is that you can see and understand it clearly, and seeing, will use your very good mind to obey these demands of nature. No matter where you live, or what your work or your hours, you can find a reasonable facsimile of all these requirements. And even though it may be a little more inconvenient for you than for people who live on a South Sea island, you are still under the demands of your body's laws.

A Right Royal Preparation

Few of us can carry our necessities with us as I was told the royal family of Afghanistan did when they arrived in New York and took over a whole floor of the Waldorf, in order to have their goats and geese with them. The king and his retinue would not go anywhere if they couldn't have their goat cheese, fresh and wholesome, right at hand. But, thanks to the growing desire of our supermarkets to serve us, we can get our most exotic and special requirements from them, trundle them out in those helpful metal baskets and proceed on our healthful way. Our every need is met.

Special Diets Can Be Delicious Today

Time was when a restricted diet meant a dismal, tasteless dining. Not so today! With sugar substitutes, salt substitutes and harmless vegetable oils, people on special diets eat the most delicious foods—if they stop to figure it out.

We have shown how emotions of fear, envy, *et al.*, drop poisons into the bloodstream; so it follows that if your cells are to be "clean" they must have the clean blood that comes in great part from loving and happy emotions.

BE A FRIEND TO YOURSELF

Somebody wrote a book entitled *Love or Perish*. I haven't read it, but it certainly is a great and true warning. Aside from all sentiment or moral tone, if you hate or begrudge instead of being loving and generous, you are committing slow suicide. Your worst enemies couldn't wish you anything worse!

If you want to get ahead of your enemies, the best way is to drop all the poisonous ugliness and let them see you healthy, fine-looking and focused on the things that matter. That will either melt them or burn them up.

ANDROCLES AND THE LION

If you have trouble with feelings of desire for revenge which are only too human, you couldn't do better than to read George Bernard Shaw's *Androcles and the Lion*. Besides being excellent entertainment, it holds some of the most profound struggles, humorously presented, that confront the human being. A motion picture was made some years ago of this remarkable story of the early Christians being herded, literally, toward Rome where they are to be used in the Coliseum games, thrown to lions, pitted against the animals in the arenas, etc.

Among them is a giant of a man, a convert. It gradually dawns upon this Christian band that they have nothing further to lose, so they might as well be as noisy, as annoying as they like, and do exactly as they please. The little feisty Roman captain in charge of them is much annoyed by their singing. They only sing the louder. Their lives are already forfeit—so what!

At one point, the little Roman soldier, in conversation with the giant peasant, says leeringly, "I understand that you Christians, when you are struck on one cheek, are supposed to turn the other. Is that correct?" The huge man admits that this is so. Standing up on something, the little soldier strikes him a smart blow on one cheek, gets down and sneeringly awaits the outcome.

The giant's hands twitch. He could crush this little upstart between them. He closes his eyes in an effort to control himself. Whatever it may cost him, he realizes that Christianity is, in a sense, on trial before these Romans. The muscles twitch in his jaws. You see him praying for strength to compel himself into the Christian reaction. The outraged animal within him almost wins.

Slowly, with almost imperceptible jerks, he finally manages to get his head turned offering the other cheek to the Roman. (The audience roars with laughter, at the same time admiring him.) The soldier is so amazed he forgets to strike it (if I remember correctly) and they move on. But struck or not, the victory of the giant over his animal impulses gives him a strange inner happiness and dignity. He walks on proudly, detached from the world of "an eye for an eye and a tooth for a tooth."

He has proved to himself that he need not admit the strife of the world or follow its lower patterns. Life itself was not, to him, at that moment, so precious as his soul's view of his inner domain that he could keep triumphant over the world. The audience bursts into heartfelt applause. (Did not Christ say, "I have overcome the world."?)

HIGHER EMOTIONS BRING HEALTH

The message of Christ is a practical one. The salvation it preaches is not something afar off on a someday cloud or distant reckoning. Mohammed wisely had his followers study the teachings of Jesus (Mohammedans still do so) that they might know more of the mystical truths that, transcending the ordinary rules and reactions of men, give them the benefits, strengths and freedoms of those higher planes of the soul that bring health to all. "The meek shall inherit the earth."

It is not to make you saintly, or even religious, that I bring out these points. It is to state again and again how every penetrating mind since the beginning of time has known that man must purify his emotions if he would gain health for his mind and body.

NO GRUDGE ALLOWED

He must, as the Persians had it, "Let the half-gods go, that the gods may appear." We may love most people, but hold hate and a grudge toward one person and then expect our glands to behave. They won't! No matter what the cause, or how patent the blame, we must consign the matter to God and purify our own souls to the last jot and the last tittle. Well, we can try!

SELF-DISCIPLINE, A GIANT'S JOB

St. Paul said, "Keep thine eye single and thy whole body shall be full of light." Anyone who has ever tried these disciplines knows how herculean his efforts must be in order to succeed. Shaw's giant, making his head slowly turn, is just a case in point. Self-discipline is the most challenging job on earth. I am always entertained when someone says to me, "Why you're just a Pollyanna. You are an escapist. You want an easy way. You just don't want to face the facts of life."

It is all but impossible to explain to that particular mind that his set of facts may not be the conclusive ones at all. He is not ready to admit that there are laws within laws, worlds within worlds, and that a higher court can often reverse the decision of the lower courts. He does not want to hear this.

We just have to rise above these mundane voices and keep on listening to those that would call us higher. They, too, will one day grow to the point where they will want some help and guidance out of their animal awareness. Each to his own!

TAKE THE HIGH ROAD

Don't let anyone tell you that it is easy to take the high road —especially at the beginning. But, if you can hold to your ideals until you have achieved one or two victories, you begin to find that you are gathering force and each step thereafter becomes easier. Then, the higher you go, the easier it is.

THE VIEW IS BETTER AT THE TOP

Is not this so in all life? The higher you go, the easier it is. The most difficult feat financially is to save that first thousand dollars. In driving an automobile, we know that it takes a great deal of gasoline to start the car from a dead stop, and that the car must be in a low gear. Yet once moving and gathering momentum, the car runs faster, more freely, in higher gears, *on far less gasoline.* The higher you go, the easier it becomes. "To him that hath is given." It is a law of life, of motion, of money, of gasoline, or anything else. Certainly it is true of a talent. With skill and devotion, results, recognition and further opportunity open up before one.

These truths should deepen our resolve to pay the price of self-discipline in all the ways we seek personal victory. How does it touch or affect your energy? Listen! Listen to this wisdom, these words from the Old Testament:

> Isaiah 40-31—But they that wait upon the Lord (the law, or how things rightfully should go) shall renew their strength. They shall mount up with wings as eagles; they shall run, and not be weary; and they shall walk, and not faint.

The law will deal with vengeance; we should "wait upon the Lord." Study that!

The young body has not, as yet, been slowed down by accumulated negativities. Therefore, if you want a young body, you must set aside the weights of disillusion, despair, cynicism, disappointment, envy, revenge, and "the knowledge of good and evil." These are the demerits that banish us from our pristine Garden of Eden. Why do we gather them? That is unanswerable. But if we do not put them aside, that is unforgivable. That is to say, the law which you have set against yourself naturally works against you. But you can change your position and get over on the clean, new, creative side. "A man's enemies are those of his own house." It comes as a great surprise to many people that we are destroyed from within, not without. The Roman Empire decayed from within. Barring wars and great catastrophes, the slow processes of disintegration reach us because we cooperate with them!

A subtle fact is that the law of disintegration is not necessarily an evil one. Don't forget that our mistakes are also blotted out by it. Our enemies are also subject to it. This stream of *change* forces us to build anew—and, if we are wise, to build better.

There is much to salvage from the old structure, if we choose from it fastidiously and are willing to leave the real junk behind.

CHOOSE WELL THE FOODS FOR YOUR BODY

In a market, your eye travels fastidiously to the best, firmest, crispest heads of lettuce. You select the plumpest, tenderest string beans, the yellowest, ripest squash. Look at the sheer perfection of fully-matured grapes with their gorgeous colors! Well-arranged vegetables and fruits are very beautiful; in fact, they make artistic decorations for your house. The French use them together, often with flowers. All this lavish beauty is nature's gift to man—offering him the finest products for his pleasure and his health.

THE EMBRYO

The Chinese believe there is much extra good in immature produce, such as bean sprouts and the tender peas just beginning to form in their sweet pods, which they use whole. I have a friend who eats them raw. I must admit they are good. And there may be some virtue in eating the embryo.

It is also fashionable to add the raw China peas to the dish of chilled vegetable slivers on the living-room coffee table, which includes savory curls of white turnip, carrots and celery sticks.

VIRTUE IN SOME RAW VEGETABLES

It is surprising how many fresh raw vegetables one can get into use at the table. For instance, a package of ordinary frozen peas may be used still half-frozen by simply crumbling them into any kind of a salad. They make it delicious. Why bother to cook peas, when they are delectable raw, and so much less trouble. Following are some of my stay-young foods and ways of preparing and serving them.

A TWO-MINUTE SALAD

1 package of frozen peas, 1 can of salmon or tuna, mixed together with your favorite dressing, garnished, if you like, on top, with sliced egg. It is a whole meal, excellent at home or for a

picnic. In hot weather, it is wonderful for the middle of the day. No pots and pans to wash.

MARLENE DIETRICH COOKS AT NIGHT

My ideas are not all my own. Some of them I have invented or discovered, but many come from other people. For instance, I have copied Marlene Dietrich's way of cooking at night, and only once or twice a week. At night one is undisturbed, as a rule. Without the pressure of hurry, one adds little touches that make food unusually good. One makes truly gourmet food— and what a boon to have it ready on the following days. One can put most of it in the freezing unit, and some just in the open part of the refrigerator to be used sooner.

LARGE AMOUNTS IN ADVANCE

My mother used to cook or have cooked (down South in the summer heat) a large vessel of potatoes in their skins. These were used in many ways. First hot in chopped chives and sour cream (lacking chives, use finely chopped onions). We were all delighted when they were served to us "family fried," which meant that they were cut in very thick slices (skins on) and quickly heated and browned in a tiny bit of butter, and salted with celery salt. They could be diced and creamed, made into potato salad, and added to vegetable soup, or made into vichyssoise (which is, as you probably know, potato soup usually served chilled). And do pronounce the final "s" sound in vichyssoise.

Since cooking at home is no longer a completely feminine province, men too are interested in creating fine food with as little trouble as possible.

Choose the simpler preparations. There are many cookbooks that give ways of making many elaborate foods, but these are not for me and mine. I would rather have all that time and energy for some other pursuit, such as reading or talking to my friends. All my suggestions are toward the easier way, with just as good, and usually better, results. Some may shock the orthodox homemakers by their seemingly airy disregard for tradition. But I find most women are trying to do too many things, the hard way. For myself in self-defense, I have developed or borrowed these practices.

Try to find different things. Have you tried watercress soup, for instance? It makes a fine impression, and may be served hot or cold. Have you tried mixing pea and asparagus soup? Or asparagus and mushroom soup? A tablespoon of sherry in each plate makes it more exotic.

Serve soup in the living room from a tureen. It is convenient and chic, and makes service in the dining room easier, later on. And one certainly stays happier when one's entertaining moves along smoothly.

Even for a dinner for eight, the service at my house is buffet (after soup in the living room). The table is set, perhaps even place cards are used—but the guests go to the buffet, help themselves and find their places at the table. I find this works very well when one has only one or no maid. And the food keeps hot much longer.

Dinner for four is served already helped on four plates (in the kitchen). Dinner for six may be served that way too, or at table from dishes on a cart or shelves pulled up to the host's or hostess' right hand. If cooking or mixing is to be done at table, such as with Japanese dishes or a salad, this side table arrangement is tidier and much more efficient. Also for breakfasts where waffles or pancakes are made at table, it is best to use the side table.

A SUCCESSFUL BRUNCH

On Sunday many people invite friends home from church to join the weekend guests. Things go very smoothly, and are very appropriately simple, if on the buffet there is a hot ham (a half-ham for a few), some sand-dabs or herring on a platter, a large bowl of fruit salad, watermelon pickles, and hot biscuits with hot honey. Use the canned biscuits; they are good. Just open the package, handle lightly and spread on a cookie sheet.

No fuss and bother to mix, and the results are dependable. They bake in seven minutes. And people are delighted to have them. They always seem pleased and surprised. They are also pleased to have either honey or maple syrup served hot, so it may be poured easily from a small pitcher. Not too small; count your people.

Honey is a growing-younger food. It was believed by the ancients to possess magic qualities—and many modern people are beginning to think so too. It is completely "natural" and full of many needed elements.

Cheese of all kinds should be used generously. Not only is it a fair source of protein, but it is a product of aging, which gives rise to the bacteria we have discussed, the friendly kind. Use cheese, from Camembert to cottage. A delicious cheese dip can be made in a matter of minutes from one small glass of Rocka-Bleu cheese spread mixed with one small glass of garlic cheese spread, softened with a tablespoon of yogurt. Add a pinch of celery seed, a pinch of curry, and sweeten to taste. Loud will be the praises!

Let white bread alone. Too many nutritive elements have been refined out of it. Whole grain breads will do more for you. And try to buy the kind that states on the cover "No preservatives used." I wish it were illegal to use preservatives. They are known to be detrimental to the human body.

Use vegetable shortening, and very little of any kind.

For salads, use peanut oil, corn oil, olive oil, or any vegetable oil. At this writing, peanut oil is being greatly favored for possessing extra benefits and not having detrimental ones.

Most people have by now read somewhere that animal fats, including butter, may cause a rise in the blood cholesterol which furnishes the material that clogs the arteries. So:

Shun fat meat, or meat cooked in animal fats.

Use oleomargarine instead of butter. Few people can tell the difference these days, but your body can tell.

Use skimmed milk, because the butter-fat has been removed from it. The taste is rather flat until one gets used to it, then it seems more refreshing than whole milk. The flavor can be improved by adding a quantity of dried skimmed milk to the liquid variety, thus strengthening the taste. These milk-solids also give additional proteins and minerals, such as calcium.

Make frequent use of gelatine. It is excellent for your nerves, hair, nails, skin, and joints, and has a number of valuable elements. Learn to make delicious dishes with gelatine or the natural gelatine from meats. Chicken or sea food in aspic is attractive to the palate as well as the eye. Cold jellied consommé is very smart to serve, as is tomato Madrilene (jellied tomato juice as soup).

Use fruit for dessert as the Europeans do. If you do not have a pair of grape-scissors, write Santa Claus, for you must have them. In France, Italy and all over the Middle East, fruit is served to you on a grape-leaf, and a small fruit knife will lie with it.

Fruit mixtures are also excellent as desserts. Pineapple, a peach-half with a spoon of Cointreau, Benedictine, or Crème de Menthe in the seed-hollow is delicious—or leave out the liqueur (pronounced lick-ker, not lick-cure).

A picturesque dessert for summer is made by hollowing out a half of a watermelon and using it for a decorative bowl to contain a mixture of melons and fresh pineapple with (or without) lime sherbert. Seeded grapes are a good addition to any mixture.

Strawberries may be served in the living room as "finger food" if the stems are left on and they are placed on a tray near a small dish of cream and a dish of powdered sugar. The guest picks up a strawberry by the stem, dips it in the cream, then in the sugar, and he is protected by a tiny napkin as he conveys this heavenly morsel to his mouth.

Fresh pineapple is acceptable alone, or sprinkled with cocoanut or with any other fruit, such as seeded grapes, or even bananas.

Baked bananas make an exotic and very chic dessert. In India, and all through the Middle East and Northern Africa, they are standard. Try your skill at making them marvellous. Split the banana open and then begin with ginger, cocoanut, cocoa, vanilla, honey or whatever.

Baked grapefruit are well known in America, but many cooks do not do them well. Brown sugar, spices and a bit of wine or rum make them delicious. Serve them hot or cold.

Use your artistry, skill and gourmet interest to make your menus from natural materials. It is best to minimize the doughy things.

Learn how to cook fish. It is the test of a gourmet-cook, almost as much as a soufflé. Fish is a superb item for your growing young diet. It has many of the rich minerals from the sea that our bodies need. It is also very delicious when properly prepared. A sauce made with lemon (using a little of the grated peel too), a little oil, rosemary and oregano will bring out the delicate flavor of most fish. People who think they don't like fish have just never had it fixed in that delectable fashion. Another luring addition is sliced almonds toasted or sautéed, mixed with the sauce and put over each portion. This will make you famous among your friends. Fish once a week is not really enough for your body's needs. Eat it three or four times a week —well, twice anyway. Fish lends itself to any meal, breakfast, lunch, dinner or supper. Cultivate a taste for sea food.

Develop a catholic appetite. Cultivate a taste for everything. You should learn to like everything edible. If you permit yourself to develop food notions, you cut down your culinary experiences rather badly. Don't let yourself get to be a meat-and-potatoes eater only. A man or woman of the world should be able to eat anything on earth that anyone else can eat, including escargots (snails), raw oysters, of course, clams, frog-legs, poi, and, if necessary, rattlesnake meat. Then, one is ready to visit anywhere in the world, and be a roving ambassador.

Eat the native food. Nothing endears a traveller so much to his hosts in any land as to see him relish their native food, which is, of course, exotic to him. But there is more good will in a good appetite in a foreign land than in many speeches and loans.

For a festive occasion learn how to serve the food of a foreign land at home. Chinese, Japanese, Indian, Italian, Swedish, Norwegian, or Mexican food will make a party at your house memorable. A good curry is a gastronomic and social asset. Especially if it is served with an assortment of condiments (six, at least) usually used by the East Indians.

As a steady diet, I am sure the average American could not stand a heavy curry. But once in a while it comes as a delicious delight, a cleanser and even as a healer. More than once, when I had a cold, I have gone to an Indian restaurant and ordered an especially strong curry, which "burned" my cold away, or so it seemed. The next day I would be well.

A curry at home should be made with any meat and plenty of mixed fruits and almonds. I serve mine with a huge ring of saffron-colored rice, a platter of asparagus, an avocado salad in aspic and the condiments. It is an easily digested and not a fattening menu. It can be prepared almost entirely the day before your party, so that you are rested and ready for your guests.

If you want to be popular in a foreign country, learn to like their food, dance their dances, and, if you possibly can, speak a little of their language. But pleasure in eating requires few words! And there is infinite flattery in it, for each dish is the artful result of someone's caring. And most good food is regional. All of us like appreciation. To walk into a foreign restaurant and say, "What do you have that I can eat?" is an insult all too frequently given by Americans, I am sorry to say.

All tastes are cultivated. Children should not be indulged in their dislikes of certain foods. Most such dislikes are picked up in an attempt to copy an oldster who should have his mouth washed out with soap when he says "I don't like that." *All* tastes are cultivated. No taste is "natural." You weren't born liking beefsteak and French fried potatoes. You let this preference grow on you—and your body is suffering from lack of the elements in other foods, and one day will let you know it with a bang!

I am grateful to my mother and father, who through many stormy sessions with my stubborn determination not to eat what I didn't "like," compelled me to conquer my distaste of much good food. Today, I am no problem to a hostess, a maître d'hôtel, or a steward. My tolerance is completely catholic.

Many times I have silently said, "Thank you, Mother. Thank you, Father, for making me accept the wide world of foods. You did me a tremendous favor."

Like everything—if you can. Much energy is expended needlessly in trying to pick one's way through a menu to find something palatable. You feel relaxed, worldly, chic when your "musts" are non-existent and every meal an adventure. You feel young. Truly I know of nothing that makes us look "older" than that expression of mild distaste with which middle-aged people scan a menu. The mouth curls ever so little as though the odor of the rejected items had already reached their oversensitive nostrils. It is anything but becoming or endearing.

A young attitude would show curiosity, interest, even eagerness—smiles, obvious experience, and enthusiasm. The young point of view is never blasé. As a matter of fact, it is very passé to be blasé. It isn't chic today. It is second rate, affected only by those who haven't noticed that it went out of style with the last dodo.

A blunted enthusiasm is a loss of energy and freshness. And there is no way to make the body understand that it is an intellectual conclusion, a discriminating procedure, and therefore, in some weird way, superior. Your body says, "Why did you take that enlivening impulse away from me? Now, I shall have to be as dull and unresponsive as your ideas."

Don't ruin your vitamins. For those who wish to know the minute reactions of body chemicals, I suggest a study of vitamins. It is common knowledge that B_1 is the vitamin of courage, aplomb, and a feeling of well-being. It is not common knowledge that the emotions of sadness, rejection, and criticism cause a substance to be exuded from the glands that kills B_1 on contact. One may take a handful of B_1 vitamin pills and an hour later not have one active in his body if he has killed them with worry or vicious thoughts and feelings. That is why one feels so weak after a violent display of temper.

So, no matter what wonderful foods you may eat, what helpful pills you may swallow, you can still keep yourself on a downward toboggan physically with undisciplined acceptance of common thought patterns.

Wisdom comes often in strange packages. History says that Mohammed spread his religion rapidly for he and his soldiers captured vast territories and offered the people a choice of his faith or death by the sword. Naturally, most of them were converted quickly. Charles V conquered most of Europe and spread Christianity by much the same method. And here I am, trying to show you that if you aren't "converted" to self-discipline you will surely die. Oddly enough, the moral teachings are not dissimilar! Wisdom comes in strange packages—and truth is at the base of all good.

One remembers an amusing line of the Chinese butler in an old play, *Bought and Paid For.* He answers the doorbell admitting an old friend who asks him about himself. He answers, "Me Chlistian now. Got velly good job." But whether one begins as cynic or saint, he must meet the same inexorable laws of cause and effect.

But we are not, as yet, finished with our discussion of foods —and perhaps we shall never be done. Food is an ever-present interest and can be depended upon to keep a lively conversation alive when all else fails.

PROTEIN PROBLEMS

On the material side, the only repair substance is protein, we are told. We have come to believe that only meat supplies first-class protein. But what about entire populations in countries where meat is very very scarce? Proteins must be supplied to them in other foods, such as eggs, milk, beans, grains, cheese and nuts to mention a few. There are minute amounts of proteins in some vegetables, but perhaps their chief value lies in the potassium they supply. Potassium is valuable in cancer-prevention.

The Japanese rice diet has built a sturdy nation, but the Japanese are also heavy users of sea foods, and often eat certain fish raw. In any case, their diet is low in fat, and this keeps their hearts and arteries in excellent condition. It is known that our soldiers who survived Japanese prison camps came out with lowered blood-pressure, due, it is believed, to the low-fat food. We gather knowledge in strange ways, it seems.

In India there are certain cults, devoted to simple diet and inner serenity, whose adherents are said to live to incredible ages, one hundred and fifty being a normal expectancy. When time permits, I hope to join an *ashram* hidden in the mountains of India to learn of these things at first hand.

Perhaps you have heard of the new interest in vinegar. But it is not new to me. My amazing mother, who lived to be eighty-seven in perfect health and with her mind, memory and senses intact, used vinegar all her life. As a child I was embarrassed by her addiction to it. I don't know where she got the idea, but she kept beside her in her bedroom a small cut glass cruet of vinegar that sat on a cut glass tray with a spoon lying beside it. Several times during the day she would take a spoonful and look absolutely blissful as she swallowed it.

My mother insisted on vinegar. Several doctors, at different times, told her she was ruining her stomach's lining and wrecking her health. She paid no attention, saying, "I'm the only one who knows how I feel, and that vinegar does something good to me. Anyway, I like it and nobody can stop me." So mother had her vinegar, and the years passed.

In her healthy old age, how she enjoyed her food! I arranged for her to live temporarily in a "boarding home" while I went on a lecture tour. When I returned to get her, she had great news for me. She looked like the cat that swallowed the canary. At the home, a doctor visited the oldsters every day. In the study of geriatrics, it had just been found that old people should have a bit of vinegar every day between meals to help digest any proteins lying about. (Proteins are, as you probably know, digested by acids.) So the doctor had the nurse ply them with vinegar in the afternoon and after dinner.

You can imagine my mother's delight to be vindicated after more than half a century! Then one day, going through a "health food" store, I saw a book on cider vinegar, which, of course, I promptly bought. There was nothing new in it to me, but it did state that as we get older, beginning at about thirty, we may gradually lose our ability to digest fully the proteins we eat. We may eat the most expensive cuts of meat and still not get their benefit.

Are you sure? The digestive tract simply passes the lovely meat along and no real "trouble" may result, except that we think we have something which we have not. *Ergo,* the vinegar routine. As I told you in the beginning, I try *everything.* And I believe there is some value in that theory. Of course, I have my mother's experience to help convince me.

The apple is supposed to have its own magic. So think the old time New Englanders, who really believe that "an apple a day keeps the doctor away." The modern way is to use peel and all (except the core), put it in a liquefier, and drink your apple instead of eating it. A baked apple can be delicious and is a fine dietary protection from certain deficiencies in a cold winter.

In fact, baked anything is superior to the fried variety. Cook more in the oven and less on top of the stove, except for stews, pot roasts and soup. And many a pot roast is better off in the oven. Baked potatoes, corn dishes, most casseroles are simple things for the host or hostess to cook.

Beef Strogonoff can be a gourmet party dish if you labor a bit over it and make it fragrant with herbs, especially bay leaf; and it makes an excellent buffet, one-dish meal. With a delicate soup (since a Strogonoff is fairly heavy fare) and a fruit dessert, you have a well-rounded menu and not much trouble.

Use your freezer. Make your Strogonoff in the stilly night and freeze them until wanted. Make your soups in the stilly night and freeze them. Make your sea food casseroles at night and freeze them. Make stuffings at night, and also gravies. Have them ready, so your mind is free at mealtime.

So much for cooking ahead of time.

To prepare a meal just before serving. I always choose the things that require little or no preparation and leave almost no pots and pans to wash. Baked potatoes, corn on the cob and broiled steak, served with a wonderful salad, is a little-trouble meal.

Or ham steak, garnished with pineapple and/or apple sauce or apple rings, with gourmet baked beans. These beans have honey and fresh minced onions folded in just before serving. Do not cook the onions.

This is beginning to sound like a cookbook. By now, you have realized that I want you to understand how you can plan your time to be with your family or guests at mealtime. I want your face serene, your mind free and your energies high.

But I suggest one more thing very strongly. Do not advertise to your family, especially your husband, that you have prepared the dishes in advance. Some men have a baseless prejudice against frozen foods, so there is no use in bringing it to their attention unduly. One should also keep quiet about a diet. Concentrate and comment on flavors and the pleasures of eating. Say very little about what is good for them.

Learn to make a gourmet meat-loaf. Put in, besides several kinds of meats, soy beans, eggs, green peppers, celery and a little corn meal. Thus, you will have a most nourishing and delectable meat for sandwiches, as well as an extra dish at a party. Seasoned heavily with garlic, thyme and bay leaf, it will gain its own following. But don't tell anybody what is in it.

In Paris, I learned to like lentils. The French make marvellous lentil soup, and believe it or not, in the summer they serve a delicious and nourishing lentil salad. The cold boiled lentils are mixed with minced onions, dill pickle, and green peppers. In France, I almost subsisted on their marvellous soups, for a steady diet of their customary richness is not the best thing for me.

In all countries yogurt is respected. It is one of our best friends. It is refreshing, corrective and constructive. It creates proteins while it is in the digestive tract. I use it instead of sour cream for salad dressing, dips, or whatever. Many people buy the flavored variety. But I buy the simple white kind and eat it out of the jar with a spoon. Yogurt is so beneficial that it is almost synonymous with long life.

Remember, too, that papaya fruit or juice is a powerful digestant. Also try to eat many green and yellow vegetables and their juices. Don't throw away the water in which vegetables are cooked. Either add some lemon juice and drink it, or put it away to add to a soup. It contains many values.

If you have a blender, leave the skins on your fruits, cut out the core, and liquefy the apple, pear, grapes, or whatever. The pulp has many values for you. For this reason, it is better to eat oranges than merely to drink their juice. Almost every night I have sliced oranges at my bedside, cut lengthwise, and I eat them pulp and all, while I read or watch television. In this and other ways, make sure you get enough vitamin C for your blood vessels, to keep them young and strong. Most people are surprised and delighted with the beautiful and full-flavored fruits they find in Europe and in the Middle East. When you travel be sure to eat them.

At home or abroad one must find what best agrees with him. Everyone's chemistry is not the same, but it is surprising how similar we are when cultivated preferences are obviated.

We have spoken of the frequent rest as the key to almost perpetual motion. Each of us must apply any rule to his own hours and personal tolerance. No man is so busy, so pressed that he cannot give his mind a minute's rest; and this bit of release will communicate itself to his body.

A change of hours is a good thing. Do not let yourself get into an unchangeable routine for too long a time. Show me a couple who have been doing the same things at the same time for over ten years, and you will see a couple obviously older or building up to it. The reason?

Inflexibility is a stiffener, a drier-upper, a killer. Unconsciously, people who sometimes think of themselves as very broadminded will become so rigid in their timing that they begin to get rigid bodies, and never seem to realize the connection.

Do not get into a rut about anything, except possibly going to church. In all other matters, change days and hours and places around whenever possible. I know it is cliché to say that the only difference between a rut and a grave is the dimensions. But maybe someone hasn't heard it—and it is very, very true.

Invite new people to your house. Don't just play the same old foursome or whatever it is. Stretch your mind, your affections, your interests. Move the furniture around, and if you don't like it as well, move it back later.

12

❦ ❧

HOW TO MAKE
THE MOST OF YOUR TIME

THERE ARE WAYS TO STOP RUSHING, AND ACCOMPLISH MORE

Begin by taking another view of time. Walk around on the other side and look it all over. In stark truth, the only time you have is *now,* this minute. Last minute has slipped away; the next minute isn't here yet. You have one precious, clean, fresh, new, golden moment. What are you going to do with it?

You can give it further shine as it slips past you into eternity, or you can give it a dulling smudge. Which do you think will profit you more? Which will discharge your obligations to life the better? Which will give your own personal record (either here or hereafter) a better mark?

You have all the time there is—there isn't any more! "I didn't have time" is the age-old alibi for almost anything! I remember a friend who wanted to learn Spanish. His schedule of work and commuting would not allow him to attend classes. But he bought a book, two sets of records, one for home and one for his office, and engaged a secretary who could speak Spanish. The book he glanced at whenever he was waiting. (It is surprising how much time we must all spend waiting.) The records he played while he was bathing, shaving, dressing (his wife was getting breakfast), and at the office while he was eating lunch at his desk.

He enjoyed using his noontime. Not for him an hour of aimless gabbling in a restaurant! In a short time he began having

143

halting Spanish conversations with his secretary. Finally, he was using Spanish most of the time to communicate with her. Result: Spanish in a surprisingly short time—and he had not neglected any of his strict duties to embrace it! He had not robbed his family of evening time or imposed upon them in any way. Now he often lunches with Spanish-speaking friends.

Time is not always a tyrant. Think. It can be a willing servant. I know a mother, a French woman married to an American, who wanted to give her children her native tongue. She taught them to play games in French and read stories to them—easy stories that amused them and that they were able to follow. Soon they began to take turns in reading the stories, and each of them began to absorb, through sight and sound, the French language. It was then she knew she had won.

There must be time for thought, for silence, to invite one's soul. Just to fill every minute with something accomplished is to overemphasize the wrong use of time. Benjamin Franklin was almost obsessed by the idea of getting a great deal done in each passing twenty-four hours. Certainly his own accomplishments bear witness to the fact that he made excellent use of each day. "Dost thou love life? Then waste not time, for it is the stuff of life." Yet he found time for meditation, time to help others, and time for an amazing correspondence.

Efficiency's best use is to make time for pleasures, for arts, for friendship. An orderly, well-arranged time schedule does allow one to slide easily through a mountain of duties. Then there is time to read and plan for a trip, to brief oneself on the countries to be visited, or just to scan a road-map for a spin through one's own country. Or why not read a good historical novel? Make the time by planning well, and you won't feel guilty about it.

A good use of time adds to one's own inner approval. Since most of us feel inferior on the time question—and that sense of helpless inadequacy can easily communicate itself to other areas of our personalities—it becomes extremely important for us to take charge of our time. Time is a bully that has most of us "on the run." But if we turn and face him, we find he isn't too formidable. He can be conquered and made to serve our ends.

But, as with playing the piano, or public speaking, only practice makes perfect. You should:

1. DECIDE first that you are going to master time.

2. DECIDE that you are going to begin slowly and not be discouraged when it doesn't yield at once to your hopes.

3. DECIDE to take a year (more if necessary) to train your use of time.

4. DECIDE what you want to accomplish. Have three or four goals.

5. DECIDE what percentage of your time you will devote to:

   a. work
   b. study
   c. social life
   d. children

   e. civic duties
   f. charities
   g. an avocation
   h. sports or trips

6. Make a trial schedule. It will be full of flaws, but it will be very revealing.

7. DECIDE that you will not make a tyrant out of a schedule, for then time would have won this running battle with you, after all.

A schedule will show you, perhaps, that you really accomplish a great deal. (Today, people do a vast number of things, and still feel inadequate!) Or it may show you that by using it to better advantage you can rid yourself of some of your frustrations.

How Much Reading Do You Do?

A schedule will prove to you that you can tuck in many things you now wave aside as impossible. Take the matter of reading. If you learned to read more rapidly, you could get through a greater number of books. But there are many books one does not want to read fast. One wants to savor the pleasure of the ideas, the wording, the emotional impact, and to digest the writer's intent. One doesn't want to rush through all reading.

It is still a good idea to have the ability to do so, to use it when you want it, like all that horsepower in your car. One can take courses today that will speed one's ability to read. They sound like a good idea, not only for the reading, but for a stepped-up use of your mind. The more you have in your head, the more *alive* you are! Make way for books, one way or another.

Make a real effort not to seem and sound so "rushed" all the time. Make a project of getting out of the "driven" category. It is cheapening to the soul not to be in better command of our lives. One would think we were all Roman slaves, to hear us talk of what we must do. Perhaps we would actually do more if we stopped talking about how busy, how "rushed," how "driven" we are.

Why not cultivate the elegance of having more time? If we used the moments and breathless energy we put into the "driven drama" into listening to the other person, we would seem much more elegantly leisurely. Anyway, why force your exhausted-in-mind-body-and-clock self on other people? All these noisy put-puts sound like a skippy motor boat engine. They add nothing to your worth or charm.

It takes as much time to keep talking about how little (or none) of it you have as it would to do something interesting or becoming with those moments. Why not just stop and smile and breathe deeply instead? Like a rubber band, if you persist in keeping yourself (in concept) stretched to the limit, one day you will snap.

Since you came on this earth to grow and to learn how to use and control yourself and your world, why not first cut out the nonsense and then take another look around. You will see that you have many a margin in time that you can use to better advantage.

Eliminating fatigue will give you a richer feeling about time. And feeling more relaxed about time will give you more energy! How much energy we tie up in that one-way sense of hurry!

You can learn to go quickly, smoothly, gracefully, without awkward hurrying. If every coordinated move carries your body forward when you are walking, it will be deceptively swift. You will get across the street in the same time that a gasping, clomping hurrier takes to accomplish the same end. Besides which, your mind will be free to register the passing scene.

The hurrier is all tied up in himself. He pushes the world out of the way and hardly looks at it—a great loss to him. Watch a group rushing for a subway or a commuter's train, or just to cross the street at the rush hour. Each little human creature is behaving as though the world were his and other people are in his way.

What will be so world-shaking if you do not get a seat? You will be much better off standing, pulling in your abdomen, straightening your shoulders and thinking of the energy you are releasing into your body, than slumping into a seat and thinking how tired you are all the way home.

Even though you may hurry for that seat every day, it is entirely possible that it is making you more tired. You are probably more tired this year than you were last year; so running ahead of others to that seat hasn't paid off, after all. And by the same token, *if you continue to run for that seat because you're so dead tired, you will be more tired next year.*

Follow your thoughts and feelings on the subject and you will see the inevitability of it. 1. You run for the seat because you are tired, so you say. 2. Therefore you conceive and perform that pattern vociferously, definitely, clearly, every afternoon, hundreds of times a year. The law of mind, objectifying what you impress upon it, accommodates you and you suceed!

You are always a success. But at what are you succeeding? You are doing a wonderful job of being tired and planning to be more tired. Why not put that same amount of *definite, clear thinking* into something more rewarding?

If somebody beats you to a seat on a train or a bus, you really should thank him. You're much better off standing up and exercising and thinking pleasant, revivifying thoughts.

Use the time of travel to build, not to destroy. I can almost hear you protest, "But you don't know how I feel at 5:15." Yes, I do. I not only know how you feel, I know how you *will* feel next year. Why cooperate so enthusiastically with the law of "diminishing returns"? At least, oppose it; or better, ignore it, and put the law of *accruing energy* to work for yourself.

INTERESTING REWARDS

On a train in Italy, I could not get a seat, having given the one I had to a woman with two children. The conductor would not let me stand in the aisle, so I was forced to sit on my suitcase at the end of the car. A party of dignitaries boarded the train at one stop. One of them questioned my sitting where I was, and finally I was invited into a luxurious compartment. There I met Adrianne Gianturco, professor of music at the Rome Conservatory, through whom much of Rome was opened to me. We are still friends. All of which I would have missed if I had gotten my silly little seat.

When we take a wider, richer view of any situation, we enter wider, richer areas, sooner or later. Our little, selfish personal demands all too often trip us. But we never find it out. No one tells us. Life passes us by while we take such awfully good care of our little selves and never mind anyone else.

The truth is that we haven't the time to guard our own interests so closely. It is wasteful and clogs the channels of our lives. Then when we become ill through too much clogging, much time must be spent in getting us running again. The moral is: don't run to get ahead of someone else. Run, if you want to, for the sheer joy of it, to exercise your legs and your bubbling good spirits; but never, never, to get ahead of someone else.

A deeper reason is that just doing the best YOU can do is a far more civilized drive than trying to get ahead of someone else. The former smacks of attack simply to make an attack, or to get an advantage which is some other jungle-creature's loss. Surely we can scare up some higher motives.

Kipling wrote in his wonderful cliché-true poem, "IF": "If you can fill the unforgiving minute/With sixty seconds' worth of distance run/Yours is the Earth, and everything that's in it/And —what is more—you'll be a Man, my son!" The key word there. is "worth."

Certainly, we should make every minute bring us some good

thing. Even those who "just sit and think" and those who "just sit" will enjoy a profitable state *if* they wish every one else well, and are enjoying what they are doing.

Some of my own most profitable hours were spent lying on my stomach in a hammock watching ants on the ground below. The ants were interesting, even informative, but I found my own mind registering new sounds and slowly examining new ideas, or remembering bits of rhythmic verse or snatches of song. All manner of pleasurable subjects drifted in and out of my thoughts.

I reached a state of day-dreaming in which every limitation faded away. Effortlessly, quietly, slowly, the most lovely atmosphere drew around me. Gentle beauties gathered and in their saturation of my being, there was a dissolving of every strain and untoward thing.

An acceptance of this quiet assurance was so permeating, so complete, that it needed no supporting argument or reason. I was one with an inner essence. There was entire identification. I wondered if this could be approaching the plane of Jesus' consciousness when he heard the words "This is my beloved son, in whom I am well-pleased." The well-beloved son is in every man! He is, in essence, timeless. He is beyond contests, strivings and comparisons in the pure inner Being of him. In this timeless, unqualified state he not only *has* all energy; that is what he *is*.

And like all really strong beings, he can afford to be gentle. In fact he must be, for misuse of great power presages the end of it; *not* as a punishment, but because it moves him to another plane, away from the boon he has misapplied. Such thoughts help him to a better sense of values, help him to re-allocate his time and energies, help him to choose his thoughts and direct his emotions. They help him to know what is unimportant, and what is extremely important.

To a creative mind, one moment is exactly like another. One should burn this fact into his awareness. For it gives him supremacy over that dreadful witherer, regret for lost opportunities, or that sense of guilt about wasted time. Free yourself from such nonsense.

This moment, in basic truth, is as fraught with opportunity as any other that ever was, or ever will be. Take hold of this moment. Order it to your specifications. Begin to shape it toward your ideal of your life and yourself. It quivers with the vastness of its potential. It awaits your directing word.

Free yourself and everyone else from all sense of past mistakes, and the energy you will loose by this release of all damming thoughts will be sufficient for some magnificent attainment. This clean, fresh, powerful, free moment, now yours as a wondrous gift of your Creator, is your open road to great understanding, great joy and great fulfillment.

Time Is Opportunity

Opportunity is invitation. Invitation is recognition. Recognition is assertion of worth. Worth is energy. Thus we have, in oversimplified steps, the fact that TIME and ENERGY are the same thing, two ends of the same stick. Einstein knew this fact. Some of his calculations were based on this knowledge. What a great mind—what a great man we had in him!

The average man does not yet know his great debt to Einstein. He blazed trails we shall be following for millions of years. Christ liberated man by mystical knowing and tried to teach us in familiar language, which is often obscure. Einstein liberates man by calculation (equally obscure to most of us), explaining the intricate process by which he can and will reach those high states. Like Jesus, he could have said, "I have much to tell you, but you cannot bear it now."

Arrange your own time for some inward meanderings. You will come upon truths within yourself that will lift your entire organism into new gears. You will not need vacations alone, taken in lofty disdain of the family or friends. The whole object is to be able "to go within yourself" wherever you are, in Times Square during the rush-hour, during a quarrel perhaps, or while you're swimming across a club pool for the eighth time. You should be able to control your mind in a split second. The final truth is that if you can't shift that gear at any time you dictate, it isn't too much good to you.

Your inner life is the important part of you. The Bible tells us to "pray in secret," "go into the closet and shut the door." An amusing woman I know said recently that when she first heard of these things, the speaker might just as well have been talking in Choctaw Indian language. But as she began to follow in practice, the light began to dawn. She became a released, happy woman, whose laughter is truly infectious.

Time teaches us the value of the light touch. Knowledge should not make us solemn. It should give us the strength, the assurance, and the foundation sufficient to support laughter, love, play, creativity, and gentle strengths and beauties of all kinds. We are lifted out of the striving in which we had just barely enough for ourselves.

The indication of our strength lies in that which we have left over beyond our own need. How great is the significance of the story of the loaves and fishes. At the end, *after* the multitude had eaten, a number of baskets of left-over food were gathered. Such is the outpouring lavishness of the law of energy as applied to any point of need.

Transpose the use of your time. Time to listen, time to smile appreciatively or companionably, time to caress, time for the gracious gesture—these are the luxuries of life! And anyone can have them who will simply shift the time now spent in dark brooding, however fleeting, to happier themes.

My mind goes to one of the busiest women I know, Mrs. Ulysses S. Grant, the beloved Fanny of many friends and many activities. She goes from morning to late at night doing all the good she can. Sitting beside me last night at a ball, her husband, "U.S. IV," told me that he had never heard her speak ill of anyone. She and her ilk are busy accomplishing good things for ill people, underprivileged children, and the indigent old. Instead of bemoaning the "sad state of the world," these women are *doing* something about it!

It would be interesting if we had a little machine that would buzz when we were thinking destructively. If the time it buzzed could be measured, we could then have an accurate idea of how much time we had for better accomplishment. I think all of us might have a shocking surprise.

Wanting to Do Something Gives Us Greater Speed in Doing It

A man, it will be observed, can get ready to go golfing much more rapidly than he can dress to go to church, or to call on his in-laws. If the in-laws are on the calendar, he may be so absorbed in his workshop in the basement that he can scarcely find the stopping point; but if it is a golfing date he must make, he will drop his tools with a loud clatter and off he goes with steam and a smile.

I know a woman who has a maid one day a week. The rest of the time she takes care of her own cooking and cleaning. She dislikes jumping up from a lovely dinner and doing dishes. She wants to stroll into the living room for talk and music or a game. So, she does just that!

Different members of the family, when they go for drinking water later, often take a handful of dishes into the kitchen. But this woman refuses to be a slave to time. After she has been refreshed by a pleasant evening, she skims through her kitchen in "no time," as she expresses it. And often she does a bit of cooking for the next day at the same time.

She may make a jello dessert, a cold rice mold, bone lamb, chicken for a curry, or a beef Stroganoff. Doing a job when one doesn't want to may be good for the soul, but not for the job. It goes better and faster when one wants to do it.

Rubber Gloves

At home, probably the greatest inventions for time-saving are not a clock and a schedule, but a pair of rubber gloves and a carpenter's apron that hangs around the neck. The knowledge that one can do a quick job of silver-polishing, window-washing, or copper-bottom scrubbing without hurting a manicure one may have just gotten at Elizabeth Arden's (for $2.50), or a lovely dress, is a spur to action.

Many a wise husband would see to the supply if he gave it thought! (One manufacturer supplies an extra right-hand glove in the package—a real boon!) And the carpenter's apron really protects, allowing one to dress well in advance, instead of hysterically at the last minute. Besides which, the rubber gloves enable one to use snatches of time. For (protected) one doesn't mind doing one or two pieces of silver, one window, etc. in brief, snatched moments. (I learned during the last war to do one window and one object at a time.) Without the gloves one must arrange time for a huge project of cleaning.

A thoughtful wife will have more than one heavy apron and a pair of gloves that will fit husband, son or hanger-on, for many a man would fill an "unforgiving minute," if he were sure he wouldn't get himself mussed up. Readiness is indeed ALL.

How often would you do something if you had the equipment? How often would you write a good letter if you had bought those envelopes or had stamps? Wouldn't you fix that loose handle if you had a right-sized screw-driver? Or that leak in the hose if you had some plumber's black tape? Or vacuum one room upstairs if the cleaner wasn't downstairs?

Use Memorandums

Don't try to remember all the little things you should buy or do. Why tax your memory, which would give much better service to some poetry or historical facts, with a flood of small mundane matters? Write them down on a 3 x 5 file card. You can even buy colored ones and identify your memo in the bottom of a pocket or pocketbook.

Invent other ways of your own. These are just a few small hints along the lines of freeing yourself from anxieties and unpleasantness. Have you tried keeping all coats in one closet? Have you tried huge paper bags into which your waste-baskets can be emptied, eliminating the parade of baskets and consequent damage to them? The supermarket's largest ones will do.

Time is really a friend. It will work with you if you work it. It needs some managing, some directing. An old gardener of mine used to say, "Plan your work—and work your plan."

Think through how you can do two jobs at once. Everyone's life and demands are different, but there are many points in every life where two things can be accomplished at once. Use a time bell or clock, or a whistling tea kettle that will call you to consciousness when you want to use a few minutes for study or a nap. Then you won't mind becoming very engrossed in a task. Play a record of a language or a history lesson while you wash, mend, iron, shell peas, bone chicken, wash windows, or catch up on the news.

The One-Woman House

A wife and mother who is also cook, shopper, chauffeur, housekeeper and gardener, and who is expected besides to be a carefree hostess and a Cleopatra after dark, can often find no way out of the dilemma except such organization of her time, strength and talents as she herself can contrive. With all due respect and credit to the lady, she can greatly improve her situation by spending less time in panic and more in forethought. If you have a case of baked beans in your pantry, you will not be "thrown" when junior forgets to bring some home. Prepare for and against emergencies of all kinds. Use your telephone more, for finding what you need and ordering it.

A Near Miss

This last New Year's day we had a number of guests to dinner. My dinner was planned, cooked and waiting in an ice-box to be taken out and heated. A fuse blew out and something happened to the electric catch on the ice-box door. It refused to open. No electrician could be found. Fortunately I have two ice-boxes; there was turkey enough in the other one to form the base of a curry, which my daughter came out and made for me (a great success) while I did other dishes from supplies on hand. The guests did not know until afterward that there had been a near-tragedy in the culinary department. My old training in preparing ahead for any contingency (the fruit of living in the country during a war) saved me once again.

1. Never wait until the last minute. It is cheap insurance to be prepared to do things yourself in case the professionals must dissapoint you, or something unexpected arises.

2. Have a lock on your supply closet so careless fingers will not ruin your plans.

3. Buy two of all breakable things. If someone drops or spills one, you don't have to go all the way to the store again. By the same token have substitute supplies, in case something is spoiled, burns, or is dropped, or you find out your guest can't eat something.

4. Have a concealed ironing board and iron near where you dress, for quick pressing. Naturally, your own clothes will be ready well in advance, but a husband's, child's or guest's need can "throw" you if it arises at the last minute.

5. While you're listening to junior read, sit and thread a dozen needles with different colored threads. When you DO need one, what a boon to have it ready!

6. Exercise your eyes, your wrists and your feet while you talk on the telephone at home. In public, you might draw a crowd!

7. When you must stop for red-lights while driving, use that minute to push the head up on the top of the spine again; push against the steering wheel. Draw in the abdomen and hold it in until the light changes to green. On a fairly long trip home in the car, you may have from ten to fifteen minutes of exercise.

Now where are those people who do not have time to go to a gymnasium, have company, learn a language etc.? No one has more understanding and sympathy than I for the person who has a difficult time getting through a day of hundreds of requests and claims. I do not say that you can ever make it a perfectly relaxed breeze (although you might). My point is that you can do it all with better grace, better face and less effort and wear and tear on nerves by developing the habits of forethought, less objection, and more determined poise.

How about gifts? In a busy life of your own, *extras* are always presenting themselves. The need of giving gifts always comes as a surprise, though we know perfectly well that people are going to grow up and be married, and that we must give them a gift. They will always be having birthdays. So why not have a supply of wedding gifts and birthday gifts already packaged and keep them either at home or at the shop where you selected them. Many a shop gives this service. You select the gifts when you see something attractive for the price you want to pay. The gifts are set aside for you and put on your account, but you pay for them only as you use them. Why wait until you must scurry around and pay double the price for something you don't really like?

What are your constant needs? Many people do not even prepare ahead for their many recurring needs. I do not smoke, but I am constantly amazed at smokers who seem to depend upon cigarettes in order to get through a day with any degree of aplomb, and who are repeatedly without them. They look wounded, as though someone else has done this dread thing to them.

At such times, it is common practice for some other understanding smoker to get up, go out, walk six blocks, or drive a mile and a half to get these dramatically needed items. Perhaps I just don't belong to the club, but if cigarettes were that important to me, I would certainly see that I had a large supply of them. Since they seem more important than food, drink or even manners, why wouldn't one put them *first?* But no, time and again there are no cigarettes; and achieving them has all the excitement of a three-alarm fire, with the firemen sliding down the pole in split seconds, and dressing en route. Am I exaggerating? No!

Whatever is important to you, be sure you have in abundance. On a motor trip, one observes other motorists. A carful of fretful, demanding children usually belong to parents who have not provided comforts, pleasures and amusements in advance. The children have nothing to do but to sit inactive and think up all their new wants. The alternative is to fight among themselves to keep amused.

Arrange their time and attention. The well-organized, mannerly family has arranged for the children to have games, packages, running scores, and projects, and suitable small rewards for courtesies to each other or strangers. I heard one mother say, "Come over and have another piece of candy. You were so courteous in that last service-area where we stopped—

we all noticed it—thank you." In other words, forethought again channeled the children's energies and desires, at least in part. And even things bought in advance have to be doled out and dealt with wisely in an orderly, dependable manner.

Again, one's first move is to decide on plan, not panic. One must decide that an inner quiet and control will bring a better allotment of one's energies and time, in order to have more of both. The best uses of anything multiply its power!

And to paraphrase Rockefeller's "Take care of the dimes, the dollars will take care of themselves"—"Take care of the *minutes,* the *hours* will take care of themselves."

Does it not become increasingly apparent that *smoothness* in as many areas as possible not only reduces wear and tear, but actually draws many different kinds of energy? Duties that used to wear us out become sources of pleasure and amusement. Then our children, instead of draining our energies, become a source of personal force in many happy and profitable ways. *Now* is the *time* to see our lives in this brighter light.

13

〜 〜

HOW TO MAKE
NEW FRIENDS–AND KEEP OLD ONES

One needs extra energy for friendships. To have only enough of anything for oneself is to live at half-mast. *Extension* and *projection* are the key words of progress, growth, and forward evolution. (Even contemplation is a further look at an idea!)

The most cultured, advanced, travelled, informed people are usually the ones whose interest reaches the farthest. They are not to be confused with brash, pushing self-seekers who, for instance, go about on shipboard handing out their cards, and (horror of horrors), business cards, at that!

FRIENDSHIP BEGINS IN THE HEART

If you start on a trip with an honest, warm interest in others, this feeling will somehow be communicated to them, usually without words—and usually, they will react accordingly. Some travelers are afraid of meeting "the wrong people." They stay to themselves, curl up at the edges if anyone approaches them, and miss many a treasure in new acquaintances. One need not travel to find friends. These reactions will take place at home, and everywhere.

Make at least three new friends every year. The socially experienced person doesn't mind meeting new people (unless his life is a matter of dealing with mobs of them) for he is adept at making his escape when, and as, he wishes to do so. His most basic tendency is to find new gems among people as he goes about.

There are two reasons why most people want new friends:

1. *To get.* To be amused, such as by finding new talent, new attitudes, and new approaches to the world. To find attractive people to entertain. To find people who are stimulating. Everyone is a "getter" of sorts, but within the bounds of good taste, we hope.

2. *To give.* We grow inwardly, and often benefit outwardly, when we reach out to reassure some timid person. A man or woman of the world is always seeking a way to help, to lift, to strengthen, to steady, to bring out someone. Looking back on my own travels, I remember that the person who came forward to help me in any way was always a mellow, poised, experienced individual of great quality and high position.

Be selfish scientifically. To live with one's loving interest extended to others is to live at high tide. Much good usually comes of it. It is the most profitable way in the world! It is "being selfish scientifically." People who rush by without seeing the need, bent entirely on their own concerns, have usually cut themselves off from the life-giving, profitable aspects of the passing scene.

They are looking inward, and of course they see only the small supply of everything they can carry in there. The feeling develops that they are using up this supply, and therefore they must guard and husband it. Naturally, watching this inward exhaustion, they become mentally and physically weary. Then they have a "real" excuse for not reaching out. They are genuinely tired!

Interest in others is better than a cocktail. If they looked away from themselves, sent their attention outward, they would sense the largeness of the world in which they live and its energy would begin to flow to them.

Watch a man giving a beggar or a Salvation Army lassie a coin. He may have been dragging his steps before the encounter, may have felt trapped by his inner agreement to give, but now he walks away with his chin higher. For the moment, he is lord of all he surveys—and he feels that way.

Reach out to others. When you go to a party, your first impulse is to find the people who please you, for whatever reason. Presently, as soon as possible, search out the ones to whom you can contribute something. Just your attention is often the most valuable thing you can give. Make the rounds of the oldsters and the wall-flowers. Your hosts will be grateful. The room will be brightened by more animation as these quiet ones respond to you. Everybody benefits. But you will benefit most of all.

Other people "register" your sincere interest. We spoke of your attitude's communicating itself to others. This is a little-understood area of human reaction. We are willing to admit that animals respond to the genuine feelings of people, and are able to "sense" them. But somehow, most of us balk at the idea that other people can sense our thoughts and motives—not in detail, perhaps, but enough to register our basic impulses. However, if you watch for these reactions in others and in yourself, you will find that they are genuine. Some people are more sensitive than others. Some women are often more acutely aware in this area than most men. But when a man does turn his attention to these perfectly valid processes within himself, he often out-reaches any woman.

Friendships begin with deep, inner acceptances of the people we meet. If there are no little, inward red lights flashing a warning when we are with strangers, when the "hackles on the backs of our necks" are not rising in intuitive resistance, we will do well to improve the acquaintance with new people.

Birds of a feather flock together. We recognize our own sort very quickly. Regardless of geographical location, language, customs, or costumes, people of the same level of culture the world over are astonishingly similar. They have about the same physical postures and control, the same vocal intonations, the same gracious manners, expression, and inflections. It is not difficult to recognize gentle people, no matter which way their eyes slant nor what particular tint their skins may bear.

INTEREST IN A YOUNG GIRL REWARDED

One of my trips abroad was with a woman and her teen-aged daughter. It was the young girl's first crossing. We went on a

Canadian "Empress" sailing from Montreal. As one would expect, the experienced, charming "citizens of the world" were attentive to the daughter, helping her to see and know everything, enjoying her wide-eyed response. A number of self-seeking people wanted no part of this personal generosity. Then I, on the gala night, decided to give a pre-dinner party, with one end of the cocktail lounge marked off with a velvet rope.

A number of these bent-only-on-themselves people came in their evening clothes and sat close to the rope, hoping to be asked in. They had contributed nothing to my young friend and her mother, so I simply ignored them, though they were only inches away. I didn't overlook them to punish them. They just were not a part of the atmosphere of loving, outgoing interest that dominated my party. I included only those warm-hearted people who had gone out of their way, day after day and night after night, to make a young girl's first voyage a memorable one. Some of these people are still our friends.

Strickly speaking, however, shipboard or travel "friends" carry no social claim, in the real sense, on one another. Anything further springs from a mutual wish—or the invitation of the older or more established people.

I hasten to say that we must respect the wishes of people who are traveling for a quiet rest, perhaps to work at writing or to think out a personal problem. One recognizes the people whose honest wish is to be left alone. And yet, I have known a few of these, who were traveling to lessen a sorrow or to mull over problems, who were grateful, after the first few days, to be drawn into quiet company.

New Experiences, New People, Bring New Energy

In a small Vermont village, a certain woman thought she was very tired. She was, instead, bored, because "there was never anything new there." One day she was electrified to find in the *New York Times* an article written by her banker in the village. Then she discovered that he was helping a young girl in the hills develop her talent for writing. She had no idea of the creativity being exercised right under her nose.

She decided that perhaps she had a talent for painting. She

got in touch with a small gallery in New York and soon several artists came by her place to see her work. They stayed for the week-end, the happiest, she said, of her entire life. The idea occurred to her that perhaps other artists would like to come up for week-end painting.

There were so many who wanted to come that they insisted on paying her for the use of her house. Finally, she gradually developed her place into an "Art Club" and found her income greatly augmented by her profits from it. Thus, another person found her way out into the lives of others and through them found her own gifts of creativity. She made an excellent living besides.

She sat down one day and counted her friends, those people who truly wished her well, and she was overcome with joyful tears when she got to fifty! "And I live in a village," she cried. "And I'm never tired any more," she laughed, "because I have so much to do!"

One woman learns that she has a source of strength. She told me that through an unexpected happening she really came to understand how false was her tiredness. She had always wanted to paint a sunset because she thought most painted ones looked so artificial. One day, while lying down to rest from a day's work outside, she saw the sun beginning to go down in the midst of a wonderful cloud formation. She grabbed her easel and paints and hurried to a hill, where she was painting furiously when she ran out of a certain color. She rushed down the hill to a neighbor and borrowed a tube of it, ran back up the hill, and caught just the effect she wanted. Ordinarily, this would have "killed" her, but now she did not even notice her body.

She felt so good, so elated over the whole matter, that she asked several friends over to supper, and for the evening, to talk about it. Not until they were gone at about ten o'clock did she remember that she had been horribly tired, really exhausted, from the day's gardening! Yet she had been bright-eyed and buoyant for hours since then.

The secret lay, she said, in *sharing* her find, communicating her enthusiasm, basking in snaring her friends' interest, and the mutual absorption in something of great beauty. It is entirely possible that the friends, too, became inspired and drew energy from the episode.

We must understand that the energy in friendships is like rain or manna, in that everybody around gets some of it. In fact, the best kind of friend is the one who can stimulate our energies. When friends meet, then, there is a special kind of profitable exchange. When they part, each takes with him his new charge of additional force.

Power gathers around harmony, agreement, trust, full faith. We trust our friend, and thus we give him energy. He trusts us, and we are accordingly fed a bit more force. This is one of the great values in the exchange of friendships. We are enlivened by all the gathered approval of our friends. The agreeable atmosphere, the sincere caring, lend us their special potency. When our confidence in ourselves wanes, as it does from time to time, there stand our friends! No wonder Emerson wrote, "Oh, be my friend, and teach me to be thine!" And Shakespeare, in the first act of *Hamlet,* has Polonius advise the young Laertes: "The friends thou hast, and their adoption tried,/Grapple them to thy soul with hoops of steel."

KEEP YOUR FRIENDSHIPS IN REPAIR

Attention is the vital factor. People must be reassured of your interest. Calls, notes, invitations are musts. There need not be many. People at a distance must be remembered at least once a year. Special cards for a special day may be used.

A very clever girl I know sends birthday cards. Somehow she has collected the birth dates of most of her acquaintances, and thus she scatters her once-a-year attention. Other people prefer to do their whole lists at Christmas, Easter, or some other special day—or just whenever the spirit moves them. Graduations, weddings, promotions must be noted.

A Time-Saver

A busy man I know scans several news magazines and cuts out articles, cartoons, quips, or bits of gossip and puts each of them, without comment, into an envelope for a friend whose interests may be served. How quickly this is done! One must read anyway. No time is taken for letter-writing. It takes only an envelope and a postage stamp—and lo, a friend knows you have thought of him.

Entertain

No one is so poor, or so busy, or so ill (all the time) that he can't have a group of people in to tea. From a one-room attic with a tin teapot and cracked cups to a palace garden-party with dozens of waiters, the demands of friendships can be served. The most foolish thing anyone ever did is to withdraw from social contacts because of reduced income and unattractive quarters.

Make People More Important Than Your Situation at All Times

I took my cue from the Pogolottis, friends who have lived all over the world in various stages of affluence. They never stopped entertaining. Their friends would come to them, literally, *anywhere*. I have sat on the side of a bed to take my tea with them in a one-room place in New York, and I have been served champagne by them in a vast suite with decorators and caterers officiating. They now live in Mexico City and entertain both there and in a sprawling palace they have built at Ixtapan. Besides their example, I remember the stories I heard of the determined hospitality during the reconstruction in the South. So I never stopped entertaining for any cause. Whatever I had, I offered it—and to my delighted surprise, my friends came and accepted my casual estimate of every situation.

Remember that, in the end, people put the same construction that you do on your position and your life. If you carry your head high (but not too high) and attune your mind and your aim toward the lovely and worthy and fascinating things of life, you will attract to yourself a circle of worthwhile friends.

Naturally, you will have to go where there are people. In a new place, if one is utterly without connections, one may make one's way in church groups, charity groups, or special interest groups, such as riders, hikers, dancers, artists, or museum enthusiasts. One may attend lectures at clubs, universities, again churches, offer one's help to the people putting them on, and gradually make acquaintances in this way.

One must always be willing to contribute help of some kind. One must invest in life before he receives dividends. To imagine that the world is going to jump at the chance to know you just because you look well and don't use double negatives is to delude yourself.

The world is interested, at first, only in what we can give it. And this is rightfully so. It is not a cynical observation. Why should they bother with us unless we either furnish something they want very much, or provide an opportunity for them to express their ability to give to us—two ends of the same stick. In either case, knowing us gives some kind of pleasure. This is a principle we should never forget.

Every one of us, no matter how rich or famous, is a "little Tommy Tucker" who must "sing" for his supper. If we have a talent for singing, playing or reciting, well and good—we will be welcome. If we have a husband or wife or child who is especially distinguished in some way, that will be our "entrance ticket" or the "song" we sing. Perhaps we have conversational skill and can draw out other people; a hostess will gladly welcome us. But we must have *something*.

If it is wrong for people to expect something from us, then it must be wrong for us to expect a response at any point. It is not wrong, but very right. We even expect a return when we go to church. We go to worship, but in the hope, also, that a problem will be solved by divine inspiration or intercession. And what is wrong with that? Nothing. It is right for us to expect answers to our prayers, to expect a response at every point from a responsive universe.

Give the best you have wherever you can do so—and trust life. Go among people, and give whatever you have to give—money, talent, attention—and leave any return up to the law of cause and effect. In the give and take of life, we weave the webs of friendship, the fabric of warming and sustaining responses that make life wonderful. It is best all around not to plan consciously for what you want in return. Expect your return from *life* as its law operates for you, rather than from some particular group or person.

Do not try to force some particular person to be your friend. This will place you under a great, unnatural strain and make you very self-conscious. Free people from any special demand of yours, knowing that the "law" will use whom it will to respond to you. Just pour out friendliness without too much calculation. I have known individuals to heal themselves of self-consciousness by freeing other people from any special demand. Suddenly, we ourselves feel free when we have released others from any coercion. And the friendship we feel is purified of selfishness. We see more clearly because we are looking from a higher viewpoint. We feel extended into the world around us. Smallness is forgotten. Our souls expand, and with them, our personalities and our energies.

Search for extra friends whose lives and aims are different from yours. If you are a Protestant, make friends with a Catholic. If you are a Catholic, make friends with a Moslem. Politically, often our most challenging friends are those who belong to the opposite party.

Breadth of view can come only from knowing what others think. It teaches us to like the person behind the opposing opinion. A free society will live only so long as its members like one another regardless of opinions. The human element must be placed first in our hearts if we are to have friends. This is the only way the world will ever get together in harmony.

THE HUMAN VALUES

I was traveling in Germany after World War II and I was astonished by the kindness shown me. Going through city after city, levelled to rubble, I met people who did not hate me, did not blame me, but met me as a human being. I spoke no word of German and most of them no word of English. We had to talk through an interpreter. And we learned that on both sides our hearts were grieved over the sad results of violence. At Innsbruck, Austria, crowded with tourists, one woman gave me the cot in her kitchen and she slept in a folding-chair on a fire escape.

If one travels with love in the heart for people, one does not meet hate. Political leaders stir up opposing forces, but the soldiers get together and "fraternize" unless they are forcibly prevented. This is one of the inexplicable things about war. During our own War between the States, the Northern and Southern soldiers rowed back and forth across the Potomac one winter doing one another favors and exchanging needed goods! When spring came, they began shooting again!

I have been told many times that Americans are hated in this and that country. I was told, shortly after the Suez Canal trouble, that we were so hated in Egypt that it would not be safe for me to go there. But, believing in people instead of politics or policies, to Egypt I went. Never have I had so wonderful a time!

Once or twice I was asked some "needling" questions, which I answered as best I could. But I showed a keen interest in *their* way of life, *their* art and architecture, *their* revered places and practices. I gave the children pretty cards and little candies and took them to the zoo. Some of these people still write to me. I had a wonderful time in Arab countries and equally in Israel. But my interest was in their culture, not their guns; in their personal welfare, not their politics.

There will always be divisions of opinion, and people will, willingly and unwillingly, line up behind them. But every human heart has about the same hopes and aspirations. And one person's pain is as important to me as another's.

I find that sharing little physical comforts, such as an umbrella in a sudden shower, or a bar of chocolate when service on a train through the Alps is hours slow, makes friends for me and my country. Admiring the art collection of a Moroccan chieftain, or shielding a baby's eyes from the broiling sun while the burdened young mother waits in line at a railroad station in England, have begun friendships that endure. Kindly interest has a chain reaction that girdles the earth.

When the roaring, aggressive, bellowing, shooting haters have stormed across the world with their devastation, the hearts of the

people everywhere will reach out to one another—and they will
rebuild their world miraculously, with the materials at hand.
"The meek shall inherit the earth!" Most people do not want
to believe that truth, but the time will come when they will
witness it!

Friendship Is Probably the Most Important Thing in the World

It is necessary for the young to identify themselves with their
fellows. In their groping uncertainties, their impulse is to com-
bine their strengths, a very sensible urge when the conditions
are wholesome. As one gets older, how precious become our
friendships! It is in the middle years that we are often too busy,
or too tired, to do much about them. But just as we gather
property, or plan for the future with insurance, we should lay
the lines of friendship.

Anytime is the right time to begin to make friends. Many
people say, "I've wasted my opportunities—and now it's too
late." It's never too late to do any good thing! So responsive
is our wonderful universe, so exact are its laws, that they will
function for us any time we trigger them. Forget about time—
and begin! What difference does it make how long a room has
been dark if you find the electric switch and press it?

*Do not be too selective about appropriate ages in your new
friends.* Don't reject people just because they aren't your age,
whether younger or older. Train yourself and your family to
enjoy others for their personal qualities and not because they
are of a certain age. Many oldsters are gems as friends. Many
real youngsters illumine a gathering, if they are well-mannered.

The young profit greatly by being with delightful older people,
many of whom are really "timeless." The older ones are stimu-
lated and starched up by watching and hearing younger people.
The oldest civilizations are those whose family groups embrace
all ages. How picturesque is a table or a room peopled with
several ages! Our modern tendency to segregate age groups
is a great loss to all of us!

If you find it difficult to get started socially, turn your attention to the handicapped. Invite them to your place. Many physically handicapped people are brilliant, charming, and an addition to any gathering. It enlarges your own character and your social scope to include many kinds of people.

Great-heartedness is the final passport to friendship. You will always find the most worldly, experienced, and charming people paying attention to the handicapped, wherever they are found. Among them there are rich and poor, ignorant and informed, ugly and pretty; but all of them merit your attention.

"To him that hath shall be given." "Hath what?" one may ask. Great-heartedness is the thing we must *have*, for it means largeness, scope, extension of the self. You will be surprised at the treasures that will wash up on your shore, eventually, with the movement of the waves you have started long ago. Sometimes sooner!

Long-ago kindnesses return a continuing response. I am constantly astonished by the continuing return to me begun by long-ago small kindnesses. I am almost ashamed to keep on accepting them, but I take them in the spirit in which they are brought or sent.

Healthy, socially active, well-placed people need friends, too. They will see, somewhere along the line, your heart-warming activities, and one day they will want your warmth near them. It is difficult, if not impossible, to push one's way.

Remember the parable of the sun and the wind. The wind wagered the sun that he could more quickly make a man take off his overcoat. He blew and blew, but the man only clutched his coat the tighter. Then the sun tried his way. He shone and shone and sent his warmth upon the man, who relaxed, became comfortable, then, feeling no need for the protection of his coat, let it drop from his shoulders.

Warmth always wins, even though at some particular time it may seem to be unnoticed or even unwanted. Wait! Just keep on shining! But never blow or push!

The old-fashioned "you" attitude is still best. Any good book on salesmanship stresses the thought that the focus must be on the interests of the buyer. In approaching anyone, anywhere, the effective thought is, What can I do for *you?* Can I contribute something to *you?* Can I make something easier for *you?* Can I make *you* happier? Can I make *you* laugh? Can I give *you* something delicious to eat or drink? May I listen to the expression of *your* thoughts? Tell me, please, of *your* trip, *your* child, *your* boat, *your* house. May I have *your* advice? May I have *your* recipe for curry, or that magic sauce, or whatever?

A Famous Man's Technique

Gellett Burgess, the author of *The Purple Cow* and *Look Eleven Years Younger,* had literally hundreds and hundreds of friends. His techniques of getting and holding them were as transparent as a windowpane, but they worked just the same. For instance, after leaving a dinner party, he always telephoned back about the delights of the evening, and usually asked for a recipe.

I remember feeling slightly vexed that he had called me so late, and being a little annoyed at having to dig up the recipe, but before the conversation was finished, the full flattery of the whole thing had begun to take effect, and I considered him lovable!

Young, Beautiful, and Popular at Eighty-two

Mrs. L. H. Daingerfield in Los Angeles, the beloved Frances of thousands of friends, claims to be eighty-two years old. She looks perhaps sixty and shows no signs of getting older. Her flesh is smooth, soft, and practically wrinkle-free. Her eyes are bright. I've never known her to be ill. She is a very pretty woman. She goes from morning until late at night, tiring out many a younger person. Her interests lie chiefly in the musical world. She is one of the creators and continuing sponsors of the Youth Orchestra, and has unearthed much young talent. She is the friend of queens and school children. She seems to be present at every party, ball, concert, and committee meeting held in the city!

Her secret? She seldom thinks about herself. Once a week

she plans her clothes, and the rest of the time she just puts them on, though she always looks well dressed. Because people are always asking her about herself, she has a little patter she gives them. But before she has finished, her thoughts are already reaching out to something or somebody else. She is always rolling someone's logs, always working on the ball or the benefit to raise money for young artists. She loves her friends. She is always talking about their *good* qualities.

Why wouldn't she stay young and healthy? Her whole being is keyed to youth, the harmonies and rhythms of music, new beauties, talents, budding genius, the wonders and virtues of people! Certainly she has her critics, but not one of them can keep up with her. They seem to be just giving in to the old impulse to pull others down to their size. Frances just goes right on pouring out loving interest and invitations, taking note only of what is right and good in the world.

She says, "I can't afford to take inharmony, lack, and error into my mind." The question asks itself, "Can anybody afford it?" The obvious answer is: not if one wants friends—and a long life.

A Skater at Ninety

I had the pleasure of knowing the elderly Mr. Oscar Richards in the New York Skating Club when my daughter, Elizabeth, was a little girl. Sharman Douglas and her mother had put Elizabeth up for the club. The very first time we attended, I saw a man with a slender, graceful figure performing difficult feats on the ice. Then I noticed that the head on top was nearly bald. Someone told me he was the famous Mr. Richards, businessman, sportsman and philanthropist. In later conversation with him, I noticed that he brushed all old, cynical, heavy thoughts away and spoke, planned, and acted as though he were very young. He was trying to help the young skaters, trying to help organize the Ice Show for charity, advising someone about equipment. He was respected, beloved, adored. His friends were legion. His energies took him to almost a hundred years—good, vital, wonderful years!

KEEPING VERY BUSY SEEMS TO HAVE A BEARING
ON STAYING ENERGIZED

I often think of Elizabeth Arden, who is still healthy, strong and lovely. Her avid, lively mind reaches out to everything that is constructive. Her endurance is a challenge to all her friends and to all the people employed by her around the world. In addition to heading her vast enterprise, she finds the time for friends and for charity.

Among the men of our era, Churchill's durability is matched by that of Adenauer's. Of the same vintage is the irrepressible Lord Beaverbrook, who, defying his years, works at a desk at which he stands, like the bookkeepers of Dickens' time! His wisdom and experience are often drawn upon by those in even higher places. No one could be more stimulating than he. His very entrance into a room or an office sends an alerting quiver throughout the place, and everyone stands a little taller and thinks a little faster because he is there. He is rather a small man, but a giant in true dynamics. Yet no one could be more kind and hospitable than Lord Beaverbrook. Several years ago, when I was in London, he sent his car for me at the Hyde Park Hotel, and rearranged his day to entertain me at his delightful country place "Cherkley," in Surrey. His friends around the world know his unusual thoughtfulness. This proves again that the people with the tightest schedules usually can tuck in another kindly gesture!

In California, those who have the privilege are very proud of knowing Dr. Rufus von Kleinsmid, Chancellor of the University of Southern California, who, through his devotion to the interests of mankind, has become a world figure. In spite of advanced years, his step and eye are firm, his face full of light. His voice is strong and extremely effective in his brilliant oratory, which he uses to advance his ideal of international understanding and cooperation.

All of these men demand a great deal of themselves. They haven't the faintest thought of retiring. Their continuous projection of ideas into the future is one with the force they attract, generate, use and *are*.

All of us know the public figures who are popular. But I like to watch people in lesser-known groups, communities, and businesses gather the friendship of those around them, and to note how their friends enrich, illumine, and cushion their lives.

Some of the arts of friendship:

1. Bring to your friends the brightness of your life. Hold to a minimum the recitals of your woes. A little is good; too much is poison. The discipline of separating the two will teach you a great deal.

2. Roll their logs. Call on them when they're ill. Entertain for them at the slightest provocation. Never say, "Why should I? They've never done anything for me."

3. Call attention publicly and privately to their virtues. This seems to be difficult for many a man who fears he will boost someone beyond himself. The opposite is true, for constant good estimation proves that one has "a fine executive analysis of men."

Friendship is like mercy; it blesses him that gives and him that receives. It reaches past the fault and spotlights a virtue. What better thing could one do for oneself? To reject the "junk" of life and take up the thing of value is to tune one's whole being to constructive force. Then whatever the friendly gesture brings back from the recipient, sooner or later, is just an extra dividend. And if it never comes, one has already had the blessing of cleansing and harmonizing one's mind, and thus one's body. And the light shines afar, drawing into its periphery that which is like itself.

Loyalty wins. Since friendships and people's trust in you are so very essential to success in life and strength in your career, establish the reputation for speaking well of everyone. Too much criticism causes other to distrust you.

Put yourself in the listener's place. If you hear someone always pointing out the fault, spotlighting what is wrong, you know that the minute your back is turned, *you* are going to get this probing, "analytical" treatment. It doesn't endear that person to you.

But if you hear someone pointing up the virtues of others, and keeping silent about the faults, you feel that you will receive the same benign estimate when you are not present. You cannot help liking this person. You will find yourself supporting his ideas. You will back up his appointments—vote for him, if possible.

In time, you will give this person your most loving friendship. Why not build love and friendship into your life? Anything else is excess baggage. No one can do for himself all that needs to be done. We need friends. And he who would have friends must be one.

TAKE TIME OUT TO BE A FRIEND

Identify yourself with friendship and generosity. The uninhibited flow of approval between you and other people is a type of strength. If you are wise, you will find something to like in everybody, and find ways to express it.

Make a telephone call, send a congratulatory telegram, a two-line note of concern, a small gift. Carry a small address book in your pocket so that you can, in seconds, send some evidence of your concern to your growing number of friends. The small pleasures of criticism will fall away into the limbo of all worthless things; and life on affirmative principles will pay you its dividends.

So much energy is gathered from friendships that one needs only enough to "prime his pump" at the outset. It doesn't take much time to telephone someone the name of a good painter, plumber, gardener, doctor or shoemaker. Perhaps someone wants to know about a yacht basin, a sale on canned goods, a club membership, or a laundry. How much time does it take to dictate a letter to help a boy get a summer job? Or to tell your minister that his sermon was good? Or to invite a country cousin to town for a whirl?

Learn to write two or three-line notes. It is old-fashioned and exhausting to write at length every time you put pen to paper. The modern extension-of-self retains the keeping-in-touch technique but makes it possible by brevity. Occasionally, for certain friends, one sits down on a stormy night and writes twenty pages. Fine. Keep it up. But, in the meantime, do not fail to give the *pleasure of attention* to twenty or forty other people by dropping a "thought" into the post box. Each note is a friendly handclasp. Who knows but that your note to a worried friend (whom you thought was on top of the world) may save his life?

Who knows but that, years later, your traveling children may have occasion to get in touch with the receiver of one of your notes—and have a whole new world opened to them. "Though the mills of God grind slowly, yet they grind exceeding small." I have arrived at an age where I have seen the development of attention in my own life and in the lives of many of my friends.

KEEP ALL THE LINES OPEN

Do not let neglect corrode a budding friendship or stifle an old one. Declare that you *have the energy* to function with many friends. Both the declaration and the friendship itself will warm the cockles of your heart, and you will feel their inner nourishment. "Man does not live by bread alone."

Don't carry grudges. Forgive your friends. Grudges are short-circuits that seep away our energy. Everyone has, at some time, been hurt by a supposed friend. And too many people let these "disillusionments" destroy their faith in friendship. When disappointed in one person, they seem to forget the hundreds and thousands of pleasures they have enjoyed through other people, or perhaps through the same one! The whole picture gets out of balance. This is bad for the other departments of your life, too. Poisons seep around.

Do not expect to find perfect friends. When you are hurt, that is the time to sit down and make a list of all the good things about the person who has hurt you. Each of them will be a reason why you should forgive him. No one is perfect, not even you! Wouldn't you like to have *your* shortcomings, *your* lapses, overlooked? Of course you would! Then you must overlook those of your friends.

Most quarrels are based on misunderstandings or exaggerations of some kind. Wise and kind people usually measure the worth against the offense and decide to forget the latter. Two of my friends in Los Angeles have resumed a friendship cooled for several years by their focusing on each other's less attractive qualities. Both of them are grown-up enough to forget the whole thing, and now they exchange social courtesies. There is an intense relief all around, for it was often uncomfortable to invite them both to the same party, though they had many mutual friends. Harmony, or at least acceptance, now reigns. Much credit is due both of them. I don't suppose it was easy for either of them. They showed their growth, nobility, and largeness by their wiping off the old score.

There was a buzz of talk about it, but it lasted only a few minutes; and now everybody is back to a happy normal. Isn't that wonderful? Would that all of us would open the dams of disapproval and let love wash through our hearts to add to the world's sum total of *agreement*.

HAS THE THOUGHT EVER STRUCK YOU THAT WORLD DIFFICULTIES ARE JUST THE MULTIPLICATION OF OUR SMALL PERSONAL EMOTIONS ABOUT PEOPLE?

Isn't it possible that if each person healed himself of judgments and resistances, the world's inharmony would vanish into the fogs of misunderstanding from which it rose, and clarity of truthful vision would reign? How can we ever have peace involving billions of people and hundreds of nations as long as each of us lives within the confines of emotional stresses, confusions, resistances, and hostilities? Have you an enemy? Go and make your peace! Forgive your brother, sister, mother or friend. You do not have to answer for their faults. But you *do* have to answer for holding the fault on them in thought. "Loose him and let him go," said the Christ every time a man was brought before him bound. Are we binding others?

I did, as a young woman. I sat in judgment on some of my friends, considering them inferior, common. I bound their immaturity upon them in thought; and who was the loser? I, of course. A few years later, these people went past me as though I were standing still! I am repeating this story from the standpoint of the law that says:

"Whatever we hold about another person is really about ourselves."

It is *we* who are holding the faulty picture! Though it is addressed to someone else, the subconscious mind cannot read; and the faulty pattern is being worked into our lives, our affairs, our minds, and our bodies!

Only one thing is lacking. I know a woman who is beautiful, well-off, well-placed, very lovely in many ways—but she has set herself up as a judge of all who come before her. Some of her measuring sticks are just arbitrary ones, of her own choosing, and do not necessarily obtain elsewhere. This inner gathering of inharmony has expressed itself in her life as an almost unbearable tension between her and her daughter. Her husband has built up his own defenses and largely ignores what she says. She wonders what the trouble is. She goes to church devotedly. But she is inwardly puzzled that her many virtues have not brought her more happiness. We have to focus on her good points—and they are many. All of us are growing in many ways, it is to be hoped. That is the purpose of living. And if it means a change of mind once in a while, we should be brave enough to accomplish it.

A Good Way to Make Friends Is to Entertain for Someone

If you do not have a circle of friends, then give a tea, or a party, for the new schoolteacher, inviting the board of education, other members of the faculty, and the parents of students. Such a party has a "civic" air rather than a strictly "social" one. Thus you will not be "pushy" in giving it; yet you can invite people from every social level. (I have worked hard to establish a trend to "honor our teachers," for we must do something to hold the good ones we have and to attract fine people into the profession. If we begin by "honoring" them socially, it will be far easier to get more money for their salaries in order to make the field more inviting to brilliant people. We must all work at these long-range values.)

As you associate yourself with the good of our growing communities, you weave a web of value from which you draw all kinds of strength.

Never resign from public benefits. Often someone says, "I've done all that. I've exhausted myself with church work, committee work, etc., and I've stopped. I just can't give it any more." That person is pulling out of strong currents of power, and usually "rests" and takes vacations until she gets soft and develops various ailments. Her mistake lies not in taking on many civic duties, but in measuring the whole by ordinary standards of spent energy. She has tried to do the extraordinary thing by ordinary means, and thus has worn herself out.

Each advance brings more friends and more energy. Normally, each promotion in authority brings new responsibilities, and affection and respect from more people. A man or woman rises in community prestige to state and then national honors. Naturally, he gathers strength from each new extension—until he takes up the idea that he is killing himself with work. That is the beginning of the end.

Why will we not accept the fact that people give us as much (and more) than they draw out? The men and women who have digested that idea have lived and served to great age. I have already mentioned Churchill and Adenauer, but let me add the great poets Robert Frost and Carl Sandburg to those who are sustained also, by the love (strength) of their many admirers all over the earth. We soon dry up and blow away without that indescribable return from friends.

The good manners of gratitude will expand your soul—and gain friends. In the rush of your life, take time to be grateful. Write those little two-line notes of thanks for good times, attention, kindness of any kind. Keep them flowing out from your pen. Don't consult a book of etiquette to find out if and when you should write. Any time anybody does anything for you, write two lines of appreciation, at least! I use "informal" cards engraved on a good paper, not stiff cards. I have them made by the thousand. I keep a pile of them on my desk so I need reach only a few inches to draw one under my pen. I write my "thank you" notes by hand, usually.

Write soon—don't wait a week. Whenever you can't sleep, slip on your dressing gown, go to your desk, and write three or four "thank you" notes. Write them while you are waiting for someone, while your hair is drying, while "long distance" is engaged in the mysteries of producing a call for you. Want to cool off a friendship? Just wait too long with a "thank you" note.

The Magic of Gratitude

The very word connotes graciousness. Both words bring "grace" to mind. They are all akin as to root, use, and meaning. We even refer to the "Grace of God" simply because we cannot think of anything higher to say of Him. In the lexicon of religion, grace is a state of bliss, of high communion with atmospheres and benefits above our supposedly common lot.

Gratitude sets in motion a veritable clockwork of salutary procedures. It begins a chain-reaction of good. When you are grateful:

1. You agree that you have received something good in some way.

2. The pattern of good in your mind is strengthened, thus building up the vortex of your inner demand for good.

3. You have, in the specific area of your gratitude, turned your back upon ill-feeling of all sorts, thus giving your heavily burdened nerves a rest.

4. Even though you are a beneficiary, your thoughts have gone away from yourself to the benefactor, with a high-quality emotion which lifts and refines you.

5. You are aware of the concrete favor, thing or pleasure you have received. This thought builds your "groove of acceptance" of agreeable material.

6. You are appreciative of the good will which prompted the favor or gift, thus raising the level of your awareness of the friendly atmosphere coming to you.

7. Your appreciation bespeaks a virtue of the benefactor, which pleases him. It lifts from him, momentarily, any deep qualms of unworthiness he may foster.

8. Your appreciation also bespeaks the capacity of the donor. You recognize and pay tribute to his ability to give.
(Even though one may say he does not wish to be thanked for the good he does, the benefits of your appreciation are nonetheless valid and valuable to him.)

9. The practice of your acknowledging virtues in someone else takes your mind away from animalistic selfishness and lifts you one more notch from the jungle.

10. You cut a groove that, like an irrigating ditch, takes the water of refreshment and life to the thirsty roots of personality. The tree will grow, flower, and bear fruit for many years to come. Gratitude is a pact with the future.

11. The channel you create to send out your gratitude is also a way by which *returns* reach you, both spiritually and materially.

You are lifted above the more difficult laws of lower states. Your case is before a higher court, let us say, that is able to reverse the decision of the lower court. In higher states, you have more protections, more aids, more vision. You can see farther. You do not have to fight your way so strenuously. Good flows to you as you send it out. You become attuned to its rich currents.

Gratitude is an elevator that lifts your whole life. The more highly-placed a man or a woman is, the more delightful will be those little notes of *appreciation* we have discussed. The more experienced in authority one may be, the more skilled and comprehensive will be the expressed gratitude.

There are a few benighted souls who feel that gratitude is too humbling. I remember hearing a man say, "I don't owe thanks to anybody. I earned every step of my way. I worked my way through school and college. I built my own business. I run my own life. I don't owe anybody anything."

Certainly one should take pleasure in the good results of his efforts, but all of us enjoy benefits and profits we had almost nothing to do with getting. Do you keep your heart beating?

What did you do to get electrical power? Oh, you paid for it, voted for it? What good would be your money or your vote without someone's knowledge of how to deal with it and bring it to your reading lamp, your stove, your battery? Did you discover electricity in the first place? Do you know how to make a tomato or a rose?

What is the life that makes you alive? Or the mind by which you think? How many kind gestures helped you before you were able to walk or feed yourself—and after that, where did you get the food? You may have worked your way through college, but what of the teachers whose clever knowledge and talents led you into the way you should go? Could you make a sunset? Or a baby's smile? Or release atomic energy?

What did you personally do about the thousands of comforts, conveniences, and blessings that surround your daily life? It is only sane and decent to be somewhat grateful to the men and women who blazed the trails for your many benefits. And it is only just to be reverently thankful to God for having made a world we can explore so beneficially. The best answer to the one who says, "But what have I to be thankful for?" is probably "Oh, grow up!"

The effective prayer is one of thanks, rather than supplication. For if we are grateful for what we have, we open up avenues for more and more. Asking for more so constantly is to reiterate constantly our lack! God's world is here for us to grasp and use according to its laws; and one of its laws is: That which you constantly declare becomes true for you. Putting your appreciation on the word "have" instead of "have not" is turning to a sense of power.

Naturally, in the crises of our lives, the passionate prayer for deliverance is usually answered, so great, understanding, and responsive is the heart of God. And in these crises, the child-heart deep within each of us does turn to the Father, no matter how cynical may have been our "intellectual" opinions. "There are no atheists in foxholes," as you may remember, is an expression that came out of World War 1.

But we do not live in constant crisis, and we must attune our habitual thinking to the idea of growing in our awareness of the powers *we* possess. One does not refute the other. A wise person uses the strengths and advantages of every avenue.

Assume That You Have Friends

Mentally, go over the people you know, and build up the qualities in them that you admire. Minimize their faults. If you continually declare, even silently, that you have few friends, and that those you have are weak or unworthy, it causes other people to fear to be your friend. They do not wish to be identified with someone whom nobody likes; nor do they wish to join a group of obviously faulty people. Stop saying you have no attractive friends and

Claim that you have *friends.* It will be as though a light shone from you that will attract others. Create in your mind and in your daily habits the atmospheres you want in the people you attract. Soon, little responses, little bits of appreciation will begin to come to you, and one by one, doors will open. (Other live ducks will settle in the water where even a painted, wooden one floats.)

Mrs. Lyman Beecher Stowe of New York is a friend of vast numbers of people. She is a patron of the arts and befriends many struggling artists. Carveth Wells once said of her, "If you have Hilda Stowe for a friend, you don't really need another." She and her husband are greatly beloved.

In the Game of Giving Any Number Can Play

I have many friends who spend much of their time and substance giving encouragement to everyone whose life touches theirs. But everybody can give thoughtful "lifts" as they go about the business of living. These plant the seeds of loving friendships. Sometimes I do not know which is the greater blessing, to have a friend or to be one!

The whole world is hungry for approval, for affection, rich and poor alike. It becomes one's great privilege to supply some of the nutriment it craves. And when we do so, someone calls us "friend." The beauty of that word echoes down the corridors of time and kindles a happy memory whenever it comes to mind. Wouldn't you like to *be* a happy memory, as well as to *have* one? Then all the power that has gathered around that word "friend" since the beginning of time will be yours to tap.

It is an amazing fact!

14

⌒⌒

HOW TO "ENERGIZE"
THE PEOPLE AROUND YOU

ALL GREAT LEADERS ARE ABLE TO STIMULATE THE ENERGIES OF THOSE AROUND THEM

You can definitely give energy to other people, or stimulate it. It becomes necessary and/or desirable to increase the energy of your colleagues at times. Whether at home, in business, sports or the arts, it falls to the lot of each of us to be responsible for increasing the energy output of those near us. Many professions are based on this need.

EXPECTATION OF A FINE PERFORMANCE

Toscanini was said to electrify the individuals of an entire orchestra so that they would give their utmost. The secret was said to be that each man was flattered by Toscanini's obvious expectation of a fine performance. They knew the maestro's standard was high, approaching perfection. The craven among them feared his scorn. But, in the end, each player interpreted the demand for the best he had to mean that the great leader was of the private opinion that each man in the orchestra was capable of high art. Each of them rose to this belief, many of them playing as they had never played before. They strove toward the ideal. Their effort was a tribute of respect for his knowledge.

If those around you respect your knowledge and performance you can infuse them with the energy to strive higher. It is impossible to give that which one does not possess. If your own energy quotient is high, your own accuracy in some skill high, you can stimulate energy in the people whom you should inspire.

You can energize children only if they respect you. Leadership in a family is, to a degree, like leadership anywhere else. You must be able to lead. The cult of being buddy-buddy with one's children, to the extent that example and leadership are blunted, has taken its toll in our national life. By all means play games with, and spend time with, your children, but let children always know that it is a privilege to be with father and mother. Then they watch, listen and learn. Otherwise, they give no respect whatever, and end by trying to teach their parents!

Without genuine parental respect, from which the child draws energy of all kinds, he may grow up with a feeling of emptiness, without standards, without respect for authority, God's or man's. Such a person seeks only his own gratification, which never satisfies; he never makes a proper adjustment to marriage, an employer, a religion or anything else. A great percentage of such people are always tired. These are the people who seek multiple divorces, have serious breakdowns, are rootless emotionally, and, all too often, take their own lives.

Some people grow up tired because they have not been trained to respect anybody or anything. There is nothing like the presence of authority to call out our latent energies. We snap into line, correct our posture, straighten our clothes and our minds. Without it, we sink gradually into a shapeless, immature attitude that can never bring any type of satisfaction.

Let me repeat here that extremes in anything are not good. The dictatorial father, the mother who always "gets her way," (even if she has to become an invalid to do it) can make for unhappy children. But, in some ways, they are better than the "shapeless" family. Moderation in all things is naturally the better plan.

The fact remains that respect, admiration, and a sense of pride, can be a spur to energy-gaining attitudes. I do not mean that one should strive always to appear perfect to one's children. There can be discouragement in too-rigid demands.

Often a family tragedy can be the means of finding strengths. At the risk of a seeming contradiction I must say that children who have been enlisted in protecting family weaknesses often develop amazing strengths. But before they wish to shield a lack in mother or father, sister or brother, they must love and respect that person for excellence in another area.

The family that disciplines itself to stand together, to compensate for a family fault or lack, will develop many personal skills. Its members will be able to keep their tongues when they should. They will be able to have compassion for others. They will have more understanding of human nature. They will be able to have pity without destroying their own ideals. They will have some practice in several kinds of self-control.

Family life can mean combined strength. Each member of your family should feel that, added to his own powers, he enjoys the total force of all the other members. Children, particularly, take pride in possessing the "backing" of the entire household. Lacking it, they quite naturally seek security in the "gang."

Why not give them the strength of family projects, trips, picnics, games with running scores at home, painting, cleaning, organizing and just plain lolling about together? Sometimes being quiet together can bring out ideas that add to a feeling of solidarity, and create a sense of family strength.

Family projects foster energy. Have you ever noticed the pride in Johnny's face when, on Sunday, a young caller at the door asks him to come over and play? And have you noticed that pride deepen when he can say, "I'd like to, but Dad's taking us all on a jaunt this afternoon." Or, "We're going to start building a dark-room today. Why don't you stay and help us?" Thus another youngster benefits by the inspiring joining of forces.

Family fun becomes a focus of strength. Games of effort such as tugs-of-war, team play and swimming races furnish a way to siphon off the energies of the young into constructive channels. Their whole mechanism and interaction are keyed to strength, both in spending it and in training their bodies to get it and to express or store it.

But there should also be mental fun. Puzzles, the game of twenty questions, jokes, conundrums and limericks whet the mind's quickness. In pleasure, the mind leaps to clarity, thus finding answers more readily. I can never thank my parents enough for furnishing my sister and me with the stimulus of family fun. We had to write jingles and recite them, and talk on our feet on appointed subjects.

Strength of character is nurtured in games. We tried to win, but we also learned to lose gracefully. We were not allowed to cry when we lost. Sobs meant banishment, and we wanted to stay with the group. We had to step right up and congratulate the winner. When Father saw my lip quiver with self-pity, he would whisper, "It isn't the end of the world. There'll be other chances. Your sister needs to win, too. Take your turn."

Thus were planted the disciplines that enabled me to survive ill luck, grief, and those dull plateaus in every life. Thus I learned what power there is in keeping on keeping on, with the principle of life's resurgence bringing me, in the over-all picture, a myriad of satisfactions. Thus I learned that the strength of the team lies in each individual member of it. There were also gains in consideration and self-restraint.

We can energize others by calling on their strength. When we see someone tiring, sagging, on the edge of discouragement, we can reverse his feeling by asking his advice, his assistance. He sees himself through new eyes when someone thinks his judgment good, his power of decision unimpaired. I remember a disconsolate neighbor coming to my mother for comfort. Her face was red and swollen with weeping.

Find something to approve. I knew my mother was trying to think of something complimentary to say to her to start her valuing herself again. Mother's eyes quickly swept over her—and almost instantly she said, "What lovely elbows you have!" The woman was so surprised that she stopped crying, and tried to look at her elbows. In a moment both of them were laughing, the tension was broken, and the woman, with Mother's help, reassembled herself.

We can energize ourselves by finding qualities in ourselves we can like. Whenever confidence ebbs dangerously, we should go over our good points. Even one good performance or one ability is enough to cling to until we can get ourselves reorganized.

Every person should realize that he has God-given powers within him. Talents, capacities, skills, even very small ones, give us a feeling of worth, and worth is strength.

Inspire your friends by calling on their skills. Call them into action. When you have a distinguished visitor, call on your ex-mayor or your retired librarian for material for a speech of presentation. When you need the name of a sixteenth-century painter, call up a bookworm you know and ask him. When you need a fourth for bridge, ask a recluse to fill in. Many "tired" and "retired" people have much to give, are richer than they have ever been in those values that make life productive. Give them back their energies by calling upon them! And keep the young people you know from rusting by insisting on action from them.

Focus Gives Energy to Other People

I knew a man who could energize everybody present just by walking into the room with them. His presence was magnetic. It was as though he gave an overflow of good spirits. He seemed to gather the vague, scattered thoughts and feelings in the room and cause them to come to a focal point. He was keenly interested in *something* or *somebody,* and his positiveness was an instant stimulus. This man was William B. Benton of Benton and Bowles (the famous advertising agency), Senator from Connecticut and owner of Encyclopaedia Britannica.

All successful executives can produce this atmosphere.

All great leaders have this ability.

All successful parents, preachers, lovers, architects, cooks, painters, lawyers, kindergarten teachers and politicians can, in varying degrees, invoke this principle.

It is not a mysterious process. Anybody who, by full focus on some enthusiasm, can draw the attention of others to his subject, can galvanize and enlist their energies. His fire kindles others— a very simple principle. (If someone stands and looks up at a building, a crowd will soon gather to see what the looker finds so fascinating.) You can be the sort of person who infuses a room with a new force when you enter it if you, yourself, are focused on *well-being*. One must have something to give. We cannot give what we do not have available. So, if you wish to inspire, to lead, to energize, your forces must be directed toward a point of view that is energizing. It is as simple as that!

Successful doctors and nurses have a good grip on this principle. They exude confidence! They communicate their focused consideration of the patient's problem to quiet his anxiety, to let him feel that he is the center of attention, and that great knowledge and skill are being brought to bear on the problems at hand. Beyond that there is still another intangible quality that is emanated. It is the spirit of dedication, of caring. One may respect a doctor who lacks this quality, but he is never beloved.

Sustaining love gives energy to the beloved. Robert Browning seemed to be able to lend his strength to his beloved. Elizabeth was an invalid until he fell in love with her. His love, as he expressed it, gave her mental, spiritual and physical strength. He inspired her to infuse real genius into her writings. He gave her psychic stamina. He focused her tendril forces into a unit of gentle, but great, power. And then she wrote "How do I love thee? Let me count the ways!"

But what were the ways by which Robert Browning infused Elizabeth with energy? To begin with, the magic of love itself was the strongest element. No one can explain love in its entirety, but we can recognize certain component parts. Probably the most noble and powerful part of love is the urge of the lover to support the beloved without rhyme or reason. To feel that one has the complete and dedicated backing of another being, whether or not merited, earned or reciprocated, is one of the highest experiences one can have. In itself it gives the recipient a sense of worth.

Elsewhere I have written of my father's wonderful words to me: "I'm backing you blind." True, if one thinks little of oneself, the first reaction is a questioning of the mind that would give a "lowly" creature such ill-considered love. One might temporarily think the donor "down" a little. But that is only temporary. The need of support and love deep in every human heart soon ignores such pettiness and feeds avidly on approval. I remember thinking that my father was not as penetrating as I had always supposed him to be, if he believed that I was so wonderful. But I soon forgot about that first reaction in my delight that he valued me and respected me greatly.

Appreciation energizes talent. When an audience is responsive, a performer heightens his performance. I have been interested to hear Jack Paar speak of the difference in audiences on different nights of the week. He said they were affected by the weather, by political tensions, by international news, by great accidents and tragedies, and by religious seasons, such as Lent.

It follows that our ability to energize others is colored by our inner states, our weights or buoyancy. Which gives us another reason for being able to create, at will, the best moods and feelings for the best results at all times. It is entirely possible. Why should we remain victims of the winds that blow when we have sovereign ability to choose, command, and decide the emotional and other paths we take?

In the story of my life, I have told of how the extravagant appreciation of the wife of our neighborhood delicatessen owner fired my confidence and ambition. When I would go in the shop dressed in borrowed finery, she would say, "Such a fine lady! They've never seen the likes of you around here!" Walking on air, I would go out and get everything I desired! I felt adequate to anything. I would have walked into a den of lions if necessary!

Since we can energize others, why do we not more often give them this great boon? How kind we can be! And we need not be untruthful. With the added strength of psychic energizing, almost all of us would far overreach our normal performance. And if we learn how to store this type of energy, keep it available in a kind of memory-bin, we can build it up miraculously. Most of us let its steam get away and leave us as flat as, or flatter than, we were before. Unless we know how to hold it, psychic energy simply buoys us up for a time as though we were Roman candles, and then we drop to earth again, burned out and spent.

The reason energy spurts up, spends itself and is gone is because we demand that it do so. Our expectations dictate this sequence of action. We are adamant about it, as a rule. That is the way energy has always acted, we say; it DOES act that way, and it will always duplicate that action. Nothing could be further from the truth. But if you subscribe to this age-old superstition, you will be a party to its nonsense and its limitations.

Now, form the habit of gathering into your energy-memory the experience of supporting buoyancy as you go along. Though the flames of it may subside, the gathered force need not. You can transpose it into a supporting memory—a further proof of the virtue or value that set it aflame. You can cherish the feeling of consonance with power above your customary portion, as you accept yourself, and literally *bank* it, in a savings account with LIFE. One day, as you add further joys in accepting your small accuracies and tiny triumphs, you will realize that you have gathered a considerable force.

I am not young, but I still feed pleasurably on the approval that friends now dead gave me many years ago. I still have the energy they gave me by their appreciation. Does not this show us that energy does not disappear if we hold it; that it is not a matter of calories, but of "values"? And that if we gather enough of these values, we will get any calories that may be desirable for the supporting material functions?

15

⌒ ⌒

YOUR WORK:
HOW TO MAKE IT A VITAL PART
OF YOUR LIFE

THE FINEST FORM OF SELF-EXTENSION IS WORK

Since most people *must* work at something, it is important to be on good terms with your career. If you cannot like the type of work you are doing, you are resisting it for a good third, perhaps more, of your twenty-four-hour day. That much resistance is definitely not good for you. It can wreck you.

It is absolutely necessary that you like your job. This does not mean that you will stay with it all your life. If it does not provide you opportunity to express at least some of your highest capacities, you would do well either to plan extra work or prepare yourself for something different.

Find some agreeable aspects of your job. By now, you should be able to manage your mind sufficiently to be able to cause it to find some agreeable aspects of the job you now have. For you *must* gather energy as you work—and this cannot be done if you are fighting the work. Even the most dull, unrewarding, punishing kind of work has something good about it.

You will find it far more profitable to stop reminding yourself of its galling points and force yourself to list the good aspects. For, if you let the "poor" job condition your mind to fault-finding, you will simply move that unhappy state over to the next job, and you won't like that one either. Accumulated negativity will affect your home life, your health, your entire personality. You can't afford it.

192

Whatever you are doing furnishes you with some sort of mone-tary reward. You would not have taken the job if this payment was not important to you. If you chafe at the smallness of it, then turn your mind to ways you can make the job bigger, serve more, earn more right where you are by making yourself more valuable. Usually it is possible to do just that. It is not always necessary to move to get a better salary.

Front stairs or back stairs attitude. In most organizations, two pronouns are in constant use: we and they. Ask yourself this question: When you think of your firm, do you think of it as "they" or "we"? This is very important. If your answer is "they," it indicates that deep within you, you do not consider yourself a part of the official family. You have not taken the inner oath of fealty, complete loyalty to its management or ownership. There is a cleavage, a lining up of energies to support one team or the other. With "they" in your mind, you develop, almost uncon-sciously, certain resistances, criticisms, that dilute your produc-tivity, slow down your enthusiasm to give your *all* and start a little canker of resentment that can grow to fatigue, hurt and all their ugly ilk.

A Subtle Barrier

Either adopt the "we" attitude, or see about getting yourself another job. The "they" position, in the end, demeans you, for it places you in what a secretary of mine used to call the "back stairs group," those with hired-help psychology, who count only their money and their off-time; whereas, the "we" psychology places you with the official family, where you think of the health of the whole. As one of the "we," you blend into the motivations, improvements, inventions, projections almost automatically. You will think of and do the selfless things that make you a member of the "family."

Some times this change of pronoun is all that is necessary to bring one long-awaited rewards. For thoughts are things. "They" chills off the management. "We" warms them. They feel no bar-rier unless you supply it. For your own sake, even if you leave a job, you should say of it, *"We* did some fine things over there."

The matter is in your hands. Isn't it strange how, when the smoke of argument and discussion has cleared away, we can see clearly how we place ourselves at almost every point in life. The law is quite exact. There are many people who work late hours, exhaust themselves, but have the "they" attitude. The worker is still only trying to get "them" to see how devoted he is. If he could forget about that and work because "we" have to get a certain matter finished, it makes a startling difference. However, one must give "them" a little time to get used to the new "we" position. Everything takes a little time.

Even actors feel a difference in the response of an audience when they are able to make "contact" with them. If the audience becomes involved emotionally or for some reason *wants* the actor to do well, there is a blending of we and they in the resulting success that is enjoyed by everyone there.

But one should be careful not to use the word "we" to the point where it is absurd. I remember a friend in the maternity ward of a hospital, whose nurse kept saying "And now, how do we feel?" After a day and a night of this, my friend was irritated by the expression. While that nurse was off duty, the baby was born. When she returned, sure enough, she said, "And now, how do we feel?" My friend fixed her with a vacant stare and replied, "I think we just had a baby." One can make use of a word without making it a cliché.

Work is the great panacea, the great cure-all. Largely because it means activity of some sort, and focused attention. And, as always, *action* begets energy. Work is the best poultice for a broken heart, for what would otherwise be a weary and dreary period of waiting in our lives.

In a world of increasing automation, attention seems once more focused on personal workmanship. It was feared that much automation would eliminate the workman altogether, but, to our surprise, it doesn't seem to evolve that way. Handcrafts may loom once more as great luxuries. Hand-made leather objects, even lace, may not disappear off the earth as someone prophesied. Too many of our prophets reckon without the prides and urges of mankind to "make something."

Everyone enjoys creativity. No child is too small to bring his sand-pie to you and say, "Look what I made." And no man is too old, too rich, or too elegant, to take pride in a bookshelf or something more complicated that he fashioned with his own hands. The do-it-yourself vogue was based on a deep-seated urge to create, all the way from thought to paper to product. Wise is the woman who will channel the energies of her child into some kind of handcraft. And wiser still is she when her husband's excess energies are spent on building something like boats, sailable either at sea or in the bathtub.

For a man needs an audience for his craftsmanship. If she furnishes all required admiration, she need not have too much fear of other women. He has used his energy, his inventiveness, his skill. She is his voluble-with-praise audience. He need only rest in his favorite chair and puff contentedly on his pipe.

There is deep basic pride in work. When a man speaks admiringly of another man, he always tells you what this other man *does,* has done, expects to do. When speaking of his forebears, a man, with twinkling pride in his eyes, will tell you just how his great-grandfather excelled at some craft, how ingenious was his mother, how clever was his grandfather.

Why, then, one wonders, does work seem so unattractively tyrannical to so many people? One wonders if that distaste is as true as we have been led to believe. Is it not that we have copied someone else in professing a dislike for effort? And that the whole thing has snowballed for many generations? Suppose the reverse were true. Suppose we had accumulated for hundreds of years the words and feelings of a liking for work, would we not approach our tasks with more pleasure?

Tom Sawyer Tactics

When I was a youngster I used to give evenings of recitations. I was a "diseuse." For a change of pace after demanding and dramatic selections, I would give that gem of boyhood, "How Tom Sawyer Whitewashed the Fence." There may be a whole generation of readers who are not in on Tom's secret, so, knowing that his legion of devotees won't mind hearing it again, I'll describe how he did it. He was compelled, while the other boys

were free to play sand-lot baseball and other games, to put a coat
of whitewash on a large plank fence.

With his first tormentor, he established the idea that he much
preferred to spread whitewash on a board than to play silly old
ball. This was real fun. It was fascinating. Just see how it covered, how one could spread it around with a skillful flourish!
The watching lad finally got an itching hand and said, "Lemme
try it a minute."

Tom said, "I should say not. This takes a real hand. Besides,
I like it. I'm sorry if it looks selfish, but this is for me." After a
few more minutes of watching the white brush move over the
planks to the accompaniment of Tom's cheerful whistling, the
boy felt he simply had to take a turn at it. So he said, "I'll give
you my pet fish-hook for a go at it." Tom said, "Nope."

Presently there was a gang of boys all begging for a chance to
paint. Tom collected money, jackknives, fishing poles, and all
manner of loot, then lay down in the shade while the others
whitewashed the fence for him! The lesson is clear. Make it
fun!

Creativity is a reaching of the mind. The desire to create is a
mark of culture. Some anthropologist has said that the very first
time a cave-man made a line he considered decorative on his
cave wall, in that minute culture was born. He was doing something *additional,* above and beyond the gestures of survival. Not
for food, or fighting, but for pleasure, he was *making something*
he liked.

When another man stopped to wonder at the lines on the wall,
a similar urge was born in his mind. He began to decorate his
wall, too. He liked the result. He began to think of making other
beautiful things. With stone, wood and metal he began to build;
and here his creativity, his budding culture, and his energies
flowed together, and he called what he was doing HIS WORK.

To this day, any effort expended toward some particular end
we call "work." But man has long since learned that the best
combination of urge and effort is also pleasure. To many a man
his work is his very life. His wife learns that she is number two
on his list of important issues. And yet, she should not let this

knowledge curdle her romance, for, after all, he brings her and her children the rewards of his work.

It is natural for a man to enjoy his work. What he creates or accomplishes during his lifetime justifies his existence, he deeply believes. If some of it is sufficiently concrete to endure after he is gone, so much greater the satisfaction and honor!

THE CHALLENGE OF CREATION

A man of knowledge and skill is challenged by the materials and the needs all around him. As tubes of paint and a blank canvas make an artist's fingers itch, so a bridge to be built, or a needed hospital or school foment action in a builder's brain. As Beethoven, deaf to the sound of his music, nevertheless heard it in his mind, and knew his medium so well that he could write notes in such juxtaposition that they reproduced exactly what his mind heard, so all men work toward their mental patterns. This is not extraordinary. This is the way all creativity works. These are the mechanics of creation—from mental pattern to outer manifestation.

Only a few people dislike work. If you are one of this unhappy, unnatural clan, take time out to analyze your problem and to correct it. Think of the many uses of the word and you will see how much of your life relates to it.

When you were given a puzzle to amuse you as a child, you were asked if you knew how to "work" it. Any piece of puzzling machinery brings forth a similar expression. "How do you work this thing?"

Deep in our minds is acceptance of the meaning of work as the *how* of something. What steps, in proper sequence, will cause it to perform in its intended way? Thus, the *how*, the sequence, of any mechanical or chemical procedure is, at base, the story of it. Work, then, holds, basically, the *story* of a bit of creation. And, as such, is an integral part of all the movement in the universe.

Are you bored with your work? Think then of the *story* of it, the romance of it. Though you may be doing a repetitive, unimaginative job, you can, if you will put your mind to it, think out its story value, the drama of the action of it. It will pay you to do this for many reasons:

1. Your boredom will be less, for you will already be searching for interesting values in your work.

2. The energy your boredom held dammed up now begins to trickle out and into your entire self.

3. As you invest your work with a dramatic interest up to now denied it, it becomes a focal point of other subtle, gathering energies.

4. Really seeing your job now, probably for the first time, you may perceive how it can be done better. Values begin to gather around it, because you have declared an interest, a value there, and your declaration has given it new life!

An interesting life, an exciting life, begins in the mind of the person who is living it. If you say your life is dull, nobody knows better than you! It is certainly dull if that is the way you see it! You call the turns.

But, if you see it as fascinating, if you enjoy each day—the throb of motors, the movement of people, the play of lights on a wet street, the odor of coffee at the time of coffee-break—if it is a game to you, one you will sometimes lose and usually win, you will gain its values and minimize its rubs, until you will have grown to the point where you will be automatically promoted. There is gathered force in *agreement* and keen *appreciation* that wins over any so-called competition.

ONE MAN IN ROME

A man whose job was to punch holes in shoe leather for the laces, told me that he conquered any sense of monotony by thinking of the many different kinds of people who would wear the shoes. Some would go to the palaces of Italy; others would go to the farms. Some would go to sea and others take to the air. He enjoyed his little dramas so much that he became very curious about the people who might buy the shoes there in Rome.

He formed a habit of lurking around a shoestore, after hours, and watching the people who liked his shoes. He thought the shoes could be better displayed and better fitted to each purchaser. Going inside one day, he found the courage to speak of these matters to the proprietor. Within a month, he was selling shoes to these interesting people who came to the store; and within a year, he was assistant manager in charge of opening other stores. All because he refused to bow under the challenge of monotony.

He did not fight or reject monotony. He refused to recognize it at all. Instead he invested his job with drama; then, acting out the drama, he found the people he was visualizing. This man's mind was so deeply healthy that he automatically worked the law of mind the right way! He built up the possible story-values surrounding his monotonous tasks. He did not permit his mind to stop on dead point. He understood emotionally, if not intellectually, that no man is trapped in dullness if he will use his mind to invest his work with imaginative interest and drama.

It is a fairly safe guess that the people who consider their present job uninteresting will be just as restless on the next one. The reasons may be different, but isn't it clear that the job, whatever it is, is just a backdrop against which these disgruntled ones play out their little personal dramas of boredom, of devotion to "what-is-wrong"? If they would let their minds enjoy all the suggested drama around them, they would attract or create a pattern of fascinating happenings.

Which way are you thinking? Is your mind filled with the human values, the artistic effects, the interesting mechanics of the movement around you? Or do you see it as impersonal, sterile and futile, and thus boring? Which end of the telescope are you using? Are you magnifying or minimizing the benefits and fascinations?

Your attitude toward your work colors your personality. It is all very well to say we leave our work at the office. That may be true, but the inner attitudes we have built up on the job come away with us because they are part of us. It stands to reason that if you have devoted eight hours to being appreciatively imaginative, you are going to listen to your children in the evening with more keen perception, and companionable help or laughter.

If you are restless and feel like a misfit at the office, you will also feel ill at ease at home. Regardless of so-called reasons, nobody could *make* me do that to myself! I made up my mind years ago not to enthrone discord *ever*. I make obeisances only to what is good and right. Before them, I am willing to bow low.

Insist that your wife understand your work. Go over it together so that you can discuss both problems and victories with her. The happiest marriages are those in which this sharing and supporting are carried to a fine point. Some men have tried to "shield" their wives, which is a great mistake. The laciest, most fragile, little, lovely woman is never happier than when she can (in the safety of their boudoir) challenge all the dragons who bedevil her darling. Besides which, she comforts him excessively with pillows and endearments, beverages and compliments. And all the while, he is teaching her the rudiments of how she can protect herself should anything happen to him.

Both shielding a wife and "letting her have it" can be overdone. Both points of view have faults, but in the end, the least evil and the most good come from training, informing, and sharing with a wife. Mutual interests multiply energy and express themselves in harmony, as content and as romance. They create strong loyalties.

Teamwork requires more restraint, more self-discipline and forethought, but it gathers formidable strength. Even at play, when a man and wife can enjoy most games and sports together, greater values are knit into their relationship.

Some people feel that vacations should be taken alone. I can only refer to the fact that among my relatives and acquaintances, those who started single vacations were divorced five years later. It's better to work and play together, or a reasonable facsimile thereof. Energy gathers in teamwork and play.

WORK OR PLEASURE

If people enjoy their work, it becomes a pleasure. By the same token, think how hard golfers work at their game. Think of the energy expended in riding horseback, playing polo, tennis or any of the very active games. This, however, is called "play." It would seem that we are somewhat mixed up about whether we are working or playing most of the time. It seems to depend on one thing only: do you like what you are doing? For many people, a game of bridge is sheer punishment. For others it is the most satisfying delight on earth.

The word "work" is somewhat more aesthetic in the Latin languages. In French, it is *oeuvre*. In music, for instance, one can buy *Oeuvres d'Orgue* (works for the organ). *Chef d'oeuvres* are literally "works of a master" in any field. Work here is regarded in the highest creative sense. And in foods we have *hors d'oeuvres* (appetizers), probably the most familiar use of the word to Americans, which might be translated as "beyond any works," perhaps divine or heavenly morsels. In literature, we can buy "The Complete *Works* of Shakespeare."

WORK, AN ARTISTIC PRIVILEGE

In every language, there is a profound respect and understanding of work as one of the finer privileges of the human animal. In fact, doing nothing requires a kind of absorption equal to that spent in creativity. To do nothing is very laborious, tiring and boring. Meditation, in its truest sense, cannot be said to be doing nothing. It can mean a floating contemplation that is lazily moving over a serene vista of sorts, or it can mean the most vigorous, inner application of will and search. It is said that "nature abhors a vacuum," so it is likely that there are few, perhaps no points where there is complete inaction.

One has control of his mental and physical speed, but it is safe to say that areas of emptiness, of cessation of all effort are not desirable, even if possible. One's mind, however leisurely, should always be on something. We should never let go completely of the law of the universe, the movement of mind into and through matter.

Do not reject your present work. Consider it a step, a worthy step, no matter how unrewarding it seems at present. Do it with a flourish, a graceful and full enthusiasm. Never practice dullness! You might learn it too well! It might *take,* like a vaccination. Everything and everybody works; it matters not whether they know it.

Work is the movement of becoming something. Respect it! Admire it! Love it! Accept it! Employ its laws! After all, you did not invent these processes. You are heir to them. They were given you when you were born. They are yours by right—by legal right. They are your inheritance!

Take an executive attitude toward work. No matter what you are doing, you are pushing buttons of decision that trigger first one sequence of actions and then another. You can *decide* which ones you will set in operation, but you cannot create a sequence. That secret law exists only in the mind that made the universe and gave it to man. But you can *decide, select, use*—and this great privilege is called *work.* A beautiful word that should be freed from all the connations of dullness that we have carelessly let accumulate around it. Let us, you and I, shine it up, place it on high as our greatest gift, our most rewarding wealth, the world of *doing,* of selecting the sequence of action we want for our best-laid plans—and then have faith in the result of our intelligent choice. Work—what a privilege! What an honor! What an *art!*

Let who will be idle! The heartbreaking secret is that he *cannot be idle.* So long as he lives he is working! Why doesn't he do it the way he wants to, some more rewarding, immediately enriching way?

WORK IS SIMPLY THE WAY THE UNIVERSE RELEASES ITS VAST ENERGIES!

16

∿ ∿

HOW TO PUT
YOUR SUBCONSCIOUS MIND TO WORK

HOW TO USE THIS GREAT SEA OF ENERGY WHICH RESPONDS TO THE MIND OF MAN

The human being is an extraordinary creature. He extends into infinity, into the microcosm and, oppositely, the macrocosm (the worlds of the small and large). Since there are no straight lines, as we know them, in natural phenomena, one can't help wondering if these two lines meet somewhere out in space, forming the endlessness implied in the word "infinity." In any case, a circle is implied; and within it, individual consciousness arises from the supporting intelligence which pervades it, generally referred to as the subconscious mind.

The term "subconscious mind" is sometimes in favor with some scientists, but not with others, and not with any at all times. One is reminded of Mr. Lincoln's famous remark, "You can fool some of the people all the time and all the people some of the time, but you can't fool all the people all the time."

Wishing to remain completely out of these controversies, my use of the words applies to that area, or function, which seems to lie below the conscious mind and is its silent and busy partner in physical functions, in memory, in sleep and in the (again moot) extrasensory perceptions.

Let others argue. We shall regulate and enlist, so far as we can, the offices of the subconscious to our own desired ends. Whatever it is, we can certainly understand and utilize a number of its functions.

SUPPLY THE NAME YOU LIKE

If you or some friend or member of your family object to the word subconscious, just substitute the word you can accept and let it go at that. It can be described in several ways.

1. In one way it is like a great stomach or digestive function, which must accept, without objection or question, whatever the conscious mind feeds into it. This material, of heterogeneous character as a rule, is digested and its qualities built into the body and the emotional and mental areas of any individual. Were this function clearly understood, it seems obvious that most of us would make far better use of it by selecting the best available material to send into it. But do we?

2. Without conscious direction, this receiving mind apparently acts upon what has been termed the "race consciousness," meaning the sum total of all human experience that has produced man, with his uneven intellectual development and his emotions rooted in the animal kingdom. In this sense, it might be termed the parent mind, which means to see that we function well, provide ourselves with food and mates, and protect ourselves from physical dangers. This area of mind will see us through our animal cycle of birth, maturity and death, whether or not we do very much to inform ourselves further.

3. Another facet of this extraordinary jewel of awareness is that it appears to hold the folded and hidden possibilities of man's reaching discoveries, his hopes, and his potential. But this aspect of it seems to react only to disciplines and earned elevations. Without conscious demand in this area, it does not act, or show itself. We are aware of this trio of aspects of the subconscious mind. Our interest is in the first.

We shall let the future take care of itself. Our interest at the moment is in how we can, at this moment, use our knowledge of this extraordinary force or function to aid us, to bring us comfort and profit. It seems most willing to do so.

Its chief characteristics are its responsiveness and its blind acceptance of any material dumped into it.

This aspect of the subconscious brings to mind a story of a certain rich, selfish, dishonest man who died and went up to St. Peter to arrange for his domicile in the heavenly city. St. Peter was polite but not too enthusiastic. He admitted that the new-comer did indeed have a place assigned to him, and together they set out down to streets of gold to go to it. At a turn in the flower-laden, beautifully kept lane, a gorgeous estate loomed. Mr. Rich was overjoyed and said, "Just what I would have built myself." St. Peter uncomfortably explained that his house lay farther on down the road, that this particular palace was for one of his sharecroppers. Several times Mr. Rich was pleased by a place, only to find that it was not for him. They walked on. The neighborhood became less attractive and Mr. Rich's spirits began to sag. Finally, St. Peter stopped before a small, badly made hut and indicated that this was the place for the new arrival. Mr. Rich was furious. "But how can you do this to me! I am not used to any such place. How dare you!" St. Peter looked down and said deprecatingly, "I'm very sorry, sir, but it was the best we could do with the material you sent up here."

The Materials of the Soul

Our thousand and one conclusions, motives, thoughts, and aspirations, whether they be good or bad, are indeed dropped every day into the great maw of our subconscious and become aspects of ourselves. We have already explained that even thoughts directed toward another person, especially if they form a low estimate of someone, are digested and assimilated in the subconscious mind, and become a part of you. This process of acquisitive digestion goes on all the time, and not just when you are sending selected good material into your mind.

One can well imagine a bit of dialogue between a man and his subconscious mind.

Man: "I'm miserable. I ache in body and mind. I'm unhappy too. Everything is wrong! Can't you do better by me than this? This is awful!"

The subconscious mind: "Sorry, sir, I did the best I could with the material you threw my way. There was no way to get rid of your envy of your partner, or your distaste for your mother-in-law, or your hate for the man who wronged you fourteen years ago. We diluted these all we could with your donations to the Salvation Army and your gifts to your mother, though you understand you are supposed to do things like that—it's no great extra virtue. It's what you do *beyond* what is expected that counts here. We hoped you'd take Jones home from the meeting the night it rained, but you pretended you didn't see him. And that fifty cents you put in the church box wasn't much help either."

Man: "But what can I do now? Can I make amends and get out of my miseries?"

Subconscious: "Yes, of course, but you'll have to be patient. It takes a little time. You have to build up a weight of good and pure thoughts and feelings, in order to dilute and displace this mess you've been mixing in here for the last forty years!"

Man: "How shall I begin? I'll do anything!"

Subconscious: "Well, think of the proposition as a set of apothecary's scales. In the little saucer that is down now, heavy with all your miseries, as you call them, are the things you do not want. Begin to put good things in that little saucer dangling empty, high in the air. When it is filled (though I have no idea how long it will take) that side will come down. When it is heavier than the other side it will assert its domination. It is as simple as that.

"Remember any mean, critical, dark, sad thought will add to the 'bad' side. Any fine, light, trustful, happy, unselfish thought will add its weight to the 'good' side. Grim, dutiful things help a little too, but they're not nearly as heavy with virtue as they look. But don't get me wrong. They're lots better than the bad."

Man: "But isn't there forgiveness of sins? Can't I get rid of this load all at once?"

Subconscious: "Yes, indeed you can; but the conditions are difficult. You have to accept fully the proposition that in the true pattern of the Great Kingdom there is no evil. This proposition acts mercifully to blot out any 'sin' you may be carrying around. You can really get rid of the whole thing. Just set it over there on the curb with the rest of the junk. It's picked up every morning just before dawn, and eliminated."

Man: "What do you mean, eliminated?"

Subconscious: "Just that. I don't mean to be indelicate, but there is a spiritual sewage system too, a built-in eliminator for the discards which are collected and put where they can be picked up. I can see you haven't quite got the faith for it. But you will have. Be patient with yourself and keep on selecting the material you put on the scale. Now that you understand, I expect you to get rid of all your junk, your inharmony, your selfishness, your excuses, your low opinions of yourself and/or other people.

"Sweep up and put out your deep belief in sorrow and disappointment. But be sure to put something bright in their place. The new word among those who study me is 'substitution.' One should keep up with these words. They give one great chic."

Man: "Even you have your tongue in your cheek: What can you expect of me?"

Subconscious: "Well, truthfully, now that you mention it, very little. Judging by the past, of course. But then, who knows? You may snap to attention, take control of me and yourself, and who knows what may happen? This is a fast and wonderful age. Well, there you have it."

Man: "Well, not quite. What is the best way to deal with you? To make you perform?"

Subconscious: "Why, it's as plain as the nose on my, er, your face. I am, at best, a kind of cupboard of accumulations. Now, if you don't like the accumulation you have, start your own collection. Decide to gather only bits and pieces of health and well-being. Gather trifles, even hints of the things you want, as children gather bright pebbles and pretty shells on a beach. Have a few in every pocket of your mind. I think you'll enjoy it. Most people do."

Man: "That is reasonably clear; I understand substitution. It makes sense. But how do I make you serve me? How can I make you do those extra things people talk about? It would certainly be a great convenience."

Subconscious: "Well, I see the jig is up. You're going to keep at this till you find out. I may as well confess that I have to do what you tell me to do. Of course, if you don't give orders, I have to move on to the next law, which is the race-habit law. But your conscious command is higher and first in authority.

"The trick is that you have to mean what you say—and so few people do. For instance, if you tell me to wake you up at six o'clock, I listen for the degree of authority in your voice. If I hear any doubt at all, I pay no attention. Why should I bother if you don't believe in your own mastery? But if that message reaches me clear, bright, strong, chiseled in firmness and full expectation, then I *have* to get busy—it's my nature, the way I'm made. I can't help it. I *have* to call you at six o'clock.

"Collectors have names. A stamp collector is called a 'philatelist,' for instance. Let me suggest the name "bonustalist' for a collector of 'good.' It might start a vogue. People love symbols, tags."

Man: "Just answer my questions, please. How and when shall I command you?"

Subconscious: "Oh, very well. The best time is when you can quiet other mental activity—say, late at night, and early morning."

Thus man informs himself of his power.

Man's Need for Belief in Himself

One need only pick up the reins of self-management and begin to issue requests. Just before going to sleep, tell your subconscious mind to solve the problem you give it. Hand it your worry. What is the solution? What is the way out? You are quite likely to wake up with your answer. If, by any chance, you do not succeed with the first attempts, just pin your thoughts down more firmly. Understand however, that it is yourself you are training. You do not change the subconscious, which, by nature, is always responsive.

Think of the great gift of the subconscious. It holds *all* that was ever thought and the potential of all that man may think, or be, or command! We have no words to describe the unbelievable, generous, tireless blessing of it. But this enormous storehouse of possibilities, potentials, and promise is in man and he is in it! This is the medium in which he exists, the womb in which the foetus of his future is fed. Why do we not use it better? Why do we not put it to work? Why do we not develop faith in our ability to command it?

The subconscious mind is never tired. It has been estimated that man is only one-tenth a conscious being, with the remaining nine-tenths still resting in the deeper, wider race-experience, that dead-leveller, the weight of which controls us until we take individual mastery of ourselves. The great strengths of all that accumulated force are available to the conscious directives of man.

Retrain your particular area of the subconscious. Gradually throw out the dismal, ignorant, darker race-thoughts, and substitute instead those of strong, bright understanding of man's potential supremacy. All awareness is energy.

Substitute the habit patterns of all types of well-being. You are the master of your habit-mind. Rule it well. Throw out the time-worn illusion of fatigue, and demand that your subconscious mind bring up feelings of strength, endurance, well-being. Demand of it accuracy, truth, success, courage, inspiration and new ideas. You may be very much surprised at the response you will receive!

Use this extra reservoir of mind to which you have access. Be honest with yourself about what you have let accumulate in there. Let it float to the surface where you can examine it. Don't keep stuffing objectionable matter down out of sight. Get it out— really out. Face it, discard it. Command it, and the full undeniable force of the subconscious mind will back you up, will carry out your orders.

Changing your subconscious contents may be slow, but

patience works miracles. And often, sooner than you expect, your results will astonish you, as you spring-clean, discard, polish, rearrange your values and apply the arts of selectivity in the thoughts and feelings you choose from now on.

17

⚭   ⚭

HOW TO HAVE
UNLIMITED ENERGY IN THE SPACE AGE

MAN MUST LAY DOWN HIS EMOTIONAL BURDENS
AND FIND HIS INNER STRENGTH

One scarcely knows where to look! In every field, new developments are burgeoning! Science is as fascinating as a ten-ring circus, aviation is moving into the stars, and gadgets are crowding one another off the shelf. New claims on our energies assail us every day. The answer is not to "get away from it all," but to find the steam with which to ride this wonderful current of advances. It can be done!

To meet new challenges, we are being compelled to look within ourselves for the strength, even the willingness (though it has been said that they are the same thing) to live in this accelerated world.

The first thing you have to do is to make a choice. You cannot live in the old world, the pre-space world, *and* the new world that is opening up breathtakingly before you. You must throw your lot with one or the other. You cannot sustain the pace of the new world with old-fashioned beliefs, burdens and tactics. It will kill you. You had better go live in some secluded spot (if you can find one) or adjust your time, your emotions, your interests and your goals to the new world now being born.

There are those who have said that there are no more frontiers, that big business is the only way to security (either as boss or hireling), that our young people lack courage, and that the Western world is dying! There are many more of these "delight-

211

ful" estimates, but these will serve as a sample for our purposes.

Well! For a new frontier, how about the moon, or a new idea for world peace? Big business, with all its many virtues and benefits, is finally driving the world into a new evaluation of its handicrafts and gentler, more personal arts. Our young people do "sow their oats" by rebellion, which is a sign of a growing mind. But as for courage, the old spirit shows itself when really called upon. They've been bred to courage and vision. I admit it takes strange expression at times, but it is there—far, far from dead.

As for the Western world's dying, of course it's dying—everything is—but it is also being born! Scareheads and prophets of doom are a dime a dozen around any rich civilization. Only in a highly paid freedom could they criticize the status quo. But all these are good, not bad, signs. They're growing pains, signs of restless energy seeking new forms into which to pour itself. There will be only a few die-hards.

Most of us are lining up with the wonderful new world. We are eager to see what we shall find in it. And we are looking for the rulebook that may tell us how to adjust to it. We are already aware that we must make some changes.

With higher speeds, both benefits and tragedies come faster. We need almost as much emotional equilibrium to face one as the other. In sudden good fortune (a real test of taste and breeding), one must be calm and wise. In sudden tragedy, one must be calm and wise. The need is clear—emotional equilibrium. And where does one find it?

Each man must find a satisfying and sustaining philosophy— a religion he can accept. Otherwise he is dangling like a man on a rope over a precipice.

Each Man Must Find New Controls, New Self-Disciplines

My daughter has lately brought me in touch with the new-to-me world of diving, SCUBA diving. One of the most rigid demands, according to the best teachers and texts on the subject, is the "buddy-principle." In practice, it means that one does not dive alone, that divers must go two by two.

Each diver must watch the other, and if any trouble develops with one of them, the other must go to the rescue. The chief trouble would probably be with the air-equipment—the tank on each diver's back—and the diver's ability to use it. In great difficulty, both divers can use the same tank (lung). In many ways, one person can insure the safety of the other.

Now, a tank of life-giving air on one's back, and its attendant techniques, would seem to call for great presence of mind and make great demands on the principle of self-preservation. The disciplines of SCUBA diving put the other partner's safety first. A whole new set of reactions is thus brought forward, learned, ground into the reflexes.

Offhand one might say, "Well, that's all very well, but you can't tell me that when trouble comes, a diver isn't going to save himself first, last and always." Oddly enough, it isn't true. SCUBA diving, well-learned, seems to bring out the heroism latent in every breast. It thrills me to discover this truth, for it means another step away from the jungle instincts of the animal-man. It calls on the morality of man's new concept of himself as a thinking being.

The best teachers say that the whole purpose of the complicated instruction is really no more than to teach a man to *think* under water, in an alien atmosphere.

Panic, selfishness, self-preservation exist only until a diver is thoroughly trained. One learns to think rationally and morally in another world.

Another interesting slant presents itself in the diving instructions. A diver is safer if he is mannerly in the underwater world he is visiting. If he is gentle and as little intrusive as possible, his chances of living longer are much better. But if he goes kicking about destructively, roughly, he will invite retaliation from the sea creatures. How simply fascinating!

This modern craze for SCUBA diving is an interesting facet of man's good fortune in finding even in seemingly unrelated ways the training and the discipline he needs for survival. Nature works in marvellous ways to preserve her creatures. Man, being the highest one we know, has found this new way to develop an unselfish morality, to raise himself above animal panic while he is ostensibly at sport! This is only a glimpse of our new world!

New techniques for the new speeds. How vast and absolute must be our inner calm if we want to apply the new speeds without harm to ourselves! How wonderful that we have so many helpful machines and devices that cut our labors shorter! We should gradually acquire them as they come on the market. We must learn to live in our faster world, without confusion.

I recently chanced to read a survey of nation-wide traffic problems. The consensus was that our roads are not nearly so obsolete as are the drivers, who apparently have not assimilated the laws of greater speeds. The most important of these, it appears, pertains to the amount of space that should be maintained between fast-moving vehicles. There are tables of instructions for this issued by every highway department.

Motorists continue to ride on the next man's bumper, even though the allowed speed be 65 or 80 miles per hour! Men drive as they did forty years ago, the only difference being the speeds at which they hurtle over the ground.

The cure is not less speed but more obedience to the rules of physics. In many areas of our lives, we must acquire new techniques to accommodate the speeds we have and those we shall have.

High-speed motors have perfect cooling systems. Is it not equally true that a man in an authoritative post, who must get through mountains of work in any given day, would do well to keep his cooling system working well? His tempers he will throw out altogether. Instead of letting pressure make him irascible, he will have erected protections within himself, actually raising his boiling point.

Mr. Gifford, one-time president of American Telephone and Telegraph, said he taught himself one question which he always used under pressure, thus giving himself a split-second to veer away from any oncoming anger. The question was, "Now what can I do about that?"

If you want to keep your energies running in high gear, don't waste them on unimportant matters such as petty rages, confusions and emotional tailspins. The *new man* is in control of his animal responses. He stands with his feet in the animal kingdom, his heart full of compassion and pity, but his mind out in space, making the amazing (to him) discovery that "intelligence is the stuff of the gods." Intelligence is real power.

WHAT OF MAN HIMSELF?

While delving into chemistry, into metallurgy, into electronics, into principles that permit a boat to sail above the water, into the available cheap heat of heavy water, and into hundreds of other fascinating areas, man is growing more curious about himself, more eager about his personal powers. He is actually becoming willing to listen!

He knows that the scientist who says, "If you can't prove it in a test-tube it can't possibly be true," is holding his own science to limitation. People are asking, "Where is that man who said the existence of God can be proved mathematically?" They are talking about Dr. Fred Fitch of Yale, a professor of symbolic logic. They are not asking where are the men who tried to discredit the claim.

People are ready to listen to the sages of the Bible, of both the Old and New Testaments, wherein we are told of the bases of energy in the soul of man. Today science, with every move, seems to prove that the prophets of old, long in disrepute among logicians, were right after all. They are going cautiously, picking their way among the threats and superstitions that have grown up around the gems of truth about man.

They are becoming, as a consequence, more religious, not less. They are seeing their world as a matter of law, of cause and effect, animated by the choosing, selecting mind of man. Man sees himself finally as a concept of energy, and he wants to use it well.

In this world of law, cause and effect, they recognize also Einstein's "variable," which is as yet unexplained. This may be very healthy, as it is humbling for conquering man to meet inexplicable phenomena. Not everything fits into a test tube. Conjecture, logic, hypothesis and deduction can no longer say that there is no ordering power in the universe—in short, no God.

This was a popular conclusion of fifty years ago on many a campus. But today, most of the more honest, thoughtful, knowing men are saying, "It begins to look as though there were a central ordering, a force intelligently operating at the core of all life, a common denominator of pattern, which is dependable—and moral." *

In all highly developed civilizations, there always comes a movement, a cult if you will, that tries to say that it matters not how life is lived, how its functions or its pleasures are inverted, that it is each person's privilege to define right and wrong for himself. But nature's laws will not be denied. The order of the universe may not be disturbed with impunity. The purposes of nature may not be misused without setting up a nucleus for other inversions and discords. Laws are laws because they must be obeyed. Otherwise they are not laws.

And he who is lawless in any persistent way makes of himself a prey for other lawlessness, removes himself from the protections of obedience. It is he who keeps us back in the struggle to go forward. He, too, will learn.

It is not the "sinner" *per se* who presents the problem; it is the one who tries to say that his wrong way is the right way, who attempts to destroy the moral code, the fruit of millions of years of striving. He either cannot or will not see that it is impossible to destroy the moral code; he can only destroy himself, his country, his kind.

There seems to be a place in the merciful laws of life, God, and even man, for the one who does wrong and knows it is wrong, for he is a potential penitent. But for "those who defy the gods" there is only the agony of the misfit, the spiritually homeless.

We must align ourselves with the basic power of rightness. Not just because it is good, sweet or beautiful, but because it represents the quality of all true energy and strength. That from

* "Modern physicists who prefer to solve their problems without recourse to God (although this seems to become more difficult all the time) emphasize that nature mysteriously operates on mathematical principles. It is the mathematical orthodoxy of the universe that enables theorists like Einstein to predict and discover natural laws simply by the solution of equations."—*The Universe and Dr. Einstein* by Lincoln Barnett.

which we derive our lives, our minds, our being, is the pristine concept of the Creator.

While it is true that law itself does not judge its users—that heat and cold, electricity and mathematics, appears to work just as well for a criminal as for a saint—nonetheless it is true that a higher, tougher, more enduring law says there will be a breakdown somewhere in the process. For lawlessness is a breaker, and he who breaks will be broken.

Man judges himself. The mind within is clear intelligence that will not be denied. Man measures himself and judges himself. When he pretends to use new and expedient yardsticks, he knows he is fooling only himself.

THE FIELDS OF MEDICINE, PSYCHOLOGY AND PHILOSOPHY ARE DRAWING CLOSER TOGETHER

Doctors in all fields recognize the need for conditioning man for his new world, as quickly as possible. This point was brought out sharply by Dr. Menninger in a paper he read before six hundred doctors in a symposium at U.C.L.A. recently. He also implied that the *entire* man is involved in most types of neuroses, whether slight or damagingly severe. Most doctors agree that emotional habits are just that—habits; and that we can slowly train them into more comfortable and salutary patterns.

Some doctors make cautious use of drugs to hasten this ability. We have already spoken of the happier personality change in Cary Grant, the actor. The story there is that his wife, Betsy Drake, was the first to seek professional help with her difficulties in adjusting to her changed life and to his pressures.

Drs. Arthur A. Chandler and Mortimer A. Hartman are two of the helpful men who, using close supervision, employed the drug lysergic acid, diethylamide (known as LSD-25), long known and used as a stimulant by the Mexican Indians.

Dr. Hartman says that LSD is valuable in psychotherapy because "it is a psychic energizer which empties the subconscious and intensifies emotions as much as one hundred times."

Under cautious applications of thirty-one doses, Mrs. Grant

is said to have released her pent-up tangles and to have found serene balance and ease of mind. It was she who urged Mr. Grant to submit to the same treatment, with the happy results already mentioned.

Not everyone is a candidate for this therapy. The doctors have pretests that must be satisfied. They measure reactions carefully. Large doses can bring on hallucinations, whereas small ones "break down memory blocks and give release to past memories." This is extremely valuable in the many cases where the patient is remembering a past hurt and attempting to make his present associates pay for it (a factor in many divorces).

Aldous Huxley wrote a small book about his own experiences with the drug mescaline, which should warn the layman away from all such matters. All drugs which sharpen the perceptions can, under adverse conditions, bring on wild dreams. They should be employed only by the most responsible medical men.

Drugs, in some cases, cut shorter the time of struggle, and thus mercifully bring faster relief—but only when used with psychiatric therapy at the same time.

Drugs are for doctors to administer, carefully, skillfully, morally. The doctor uses them merely as an aid in carefully selected cases. The layman without skill thinks he has solved his problems, whereas he may merely be becoming an addict, his real difficulty remaining untouched, or perhaps aggravated.

In the last analysis, no matter what helps are used, man's problems are solved in the depths of his own intelligent acceptance of order and responsibility. He can usually do this for himself, without drugs, if his will to accomplish it is sufficiently strong. Remember the famous line from Shakespeare's *Julius Caesar:* "The fault, dear Brutus, is not in our stars,/But in ourselves, that we are underlings."

The will can be greatly aided by physical strength in most people. One must speedily empty his soul of discord and stress, and face his remarkable world, with its amazing responsiveness which is both flattering and dangerous. It is flattering in that little man has access to all that stupendous power; it is dangerous in that he may misuse it. Man can increase his physical strength by the proper use of his will.

Why outer space? Someone has said that man has made such a mess of earth, that it seems too bad that he is now going to scatter his greed, his neuroses and his sensuality across the reachable, inhabitable other worlds in the sky. The answer to that statement is that it may well be this challenge that will hold man's cure—which is accuracy (truth), unselfishness (the buddy-system), and altruism.

In his new world man cannot survive on the old loose thinking. In a split-second struggle with an impulse to cut corners and cheat, he can be annihilated by the accurate, swift onslaught of a power he may have unleashed.

Speed demands accuracy, toeing of the mark, hitting the center of the target—and you'd better consider the other fellow, or get smashed to bits! The time is gone when we can loll around at half-mast, satisfy our moral sense with some irresponsible mouthings, exploit other human beings, and attempt to justify ourselves by a denial of God. This burden of nonsense is today filling our mental institutions.

What we need is some surgical, incisive thinking, to train ourselves in accuracy, to revive courtesy, to respect law in all its phases. Then, we will find, to our delight and surprise, that our real inner strength is one with the Force that made and supports the entire universe. In this medium of power, which is the true nature of the self, we see vaster beauties, hear limitless melodies, feel the joy of creativity (at which sex only hints), speak with authority, and shape our world to our highest desire.

All knowledge leads to law; all law leads to morality; all morality leads to love. I do not know why *duty* (that which one should or must do) has been painted in such drab colors, for it is the door to higher states. Ignorance has done us much harm! Ignorance is our only real enemy!

Do you want to speed your world out of its discord? Then become a teacher. Not necessarily in a school, though that would be wonderful. But teach somebody what you know. Your knowledge, your experience is valuable. Do you know higher mathematics? Teach it to somebody who is lagging. Offer your services for private tutoring. Do you know how to make a heavenly soufflé? Teach it to some bride—or anybody, for that matter. (Many of my oldest friends I gained through offering my services.)

Do you want to add to your own strength quickly? Then learn something! Everything you learn is an added power, gives you another inch of mastery, releases energy. Learn a language, or how to open a can, how to give a charity ball, how to clean a mirror.

Get rid of that insane resistance to constructive criticism or suggestion. Instead, seek it! You will find a new energy and a new pleasure in using the power of other people's opinions. You, as a touch-me-not ego, are of little importance. But you as an expanding soul are about the most important thing that exists! Soul-growth is true immortality. So accept loving help.

Learn to bring out other people and you will have a crown with a star in it. Bringing out the best in others puts you high in the executive category, lifts you from any personal inferiority, and promotes you as a person. Helping others to do their best also gives you a happiness that you cannot find elsewhere.

Consideration of the other person places you in a superior position, singles you out of the crowd. The "buddy-system" in diving is a fine symbol of civilized and elevated behavior anywhere. When you give breath to a gasping person, either actually or figuratively, you suddenly realize what it means to be a human being. You graduate into the first grade above the animal kingdom. Managing your other animal impulses will seem much easier and much more desirable.

As you rise above the animal state, even by small higher attainments, you leave also its pattern of cyclic limitations and gain contact with limitless concepts. You glimpse real freedom.

You Grow as an Individual

It would profit a man to make a study of group psychology, to see wherein he is a sheep and how he may become more of an

individual, which is a basic urge of his real nature. In this area
are streams of available energy.

Dr. Gilbert Brighouse of Occidental College is very active in
industrial psychology, in which he serves the interests of employer and employee. In his own words, he does not tell them
what to do, he explains what they *are doing*—and leaves it up
to their own judgment to apply what he has said.

His findings indicate, among other things, that the employee
builds up a resentment that reaches the proportions of hate for
the paternalistic benefactor-employer over a period of time!
Unless a way can be found to make the employee feel that he
is a creator and a contributor, his deeper dignity and his
intrinsic nature is finally affronted.

Dr. Brighouse offers no solution, feeling that each employer
would have to assimilate the principle involved in his own way.
And in like manner, an employee must find his way out of cor-
roding hate. He will, then, choose his own method of becoming
a creative human being. He can begin by finding a secondary
occupation at home.

MOVEMENT IN TWO OR MORE DIRECTIONS

It would be far better for workers not to depend entirely on
the paternalistic type of big company or big government em-
ployment. If each of them had a second vocation of *his own*—
something productive he can make or do—he could tide over
slumps and periods of unemployment. Having all one's eggs in
one basket is not good. A man should *move* (work) in more
than one direction. He can do it physically, such as by having
some sort of work in his backyard, or his house after hours—
or he can invest his earnings in somebody else's work.

It is clear that if he wishes to be protected and have a share
in the world's richness of movement, he must *move*. In this way
he multiplies his earning-energy. The more movement he shares
or espouses, the richer he will become! And this would be true
no matter where or what he is—whether he deals in camels or
cargo, lettuce or literature.

One virtue of the proposed shorter business hours is that they would supply more time for a man's individual arts. Thus he could serve his innate sense of individual dignity. His energies would rise by more than one hundred per cent.

Unless we find a way to express our individuality we grow weary, tired, indifferent. When we are expressing our inward supply of pressured creative energy, we release it into our bodies, and into our careers.

Kindness, for instance, is an individual impulse; therefore, its expressions release torrents of energy. The move or feeling is strictly your own. Your avocation, your favorite sport, your rewarding child, all these release the flow of the energy of momentary self-approval. This force, linked with appropriate appreciation and humility, represents the most ideal ambience for living.

Its absence brings a weariness that causes one to think the body is spent. More often than not the fatigue you think you feel is not based on bodily states, even though you have been working, running or exerting yourself for a long time.

Physical fatigue is usually temporary and quickly corrects itself in your wonderfully resilient body. The real culprit is a personal devaluation of some kind, held long enough to empty your very soul of confidence and of its energies.

Release your body from soul-fatigue. Too often, when one is temporarily tired in body, one makes this thoughtless connection between the deeper soul weariness and the passing physical state, which literally pulls the body down. Release your body by understanding that the two types of fatigue are not the same. Your body will quickly recover buoyant energy, its natural right. Then heal your soul.

Only you can free yourself. Doctors, philosophers, psychiatrists, dietitians can only open gates, give you props, explain, coax, lure, push and pull. You, and you alone, can free yourself from fatigue. Medicine, drugs, advice, all are good if they hold you up while you find your way. But eventually you must face the point at which *you* choose, select, demand and expect a life of energy in a world of energy, motivated by mind which *is* energy.

GET READY FOR MORE SPEED AND MORE DEMANDS FOR ADJUSTMENT

We are being catapulted into new opportunities. We must re-evaluate our former concerns. We must be brave, resilient and buoyant enough to rise above pettiness that we may have thought important before. It seems impossible for us, at this moment, to solve the myriad problems that weigh upon us. But:

We have recourse to the technique of rising above difficulty. To a small animal, a mountain appears as a huge, blocking, formidable, inmovable mass. To an eagle, it is his home. He spreads his wings and is quickly above the rough terrain. It probably looks flat to him. One's mind echoes the biblical "They shall mount up with wings, as eagles." Rise in consciousness and look back on your problems. They are neither frightening nor very tall. They look simpler, fixable, solvable—and they are.

Take a look around from that height and get used to the atmosphere of space, distance, power—inwardly and outwardly—for this is going to be your "natural" world. Petty discords, imagined weakness will fall away, and you will be in possession of your natural powers, the gift of God, your maker.

The sovereignty of your power of choice is the great miracle of your being. It is greater than discoveries in electronics, space or whatever. Use it well, with compassion, courtesy and humility. With its proper use, you will become a person who can live safely in the fast-moving world of today and the faster one of tomorrow, with comfort, extended harmony and service—and a happiness unknown to the animal-man.

18

～ ～

YOU HAVE ENERGY TO BURN— BURN IT!

AND BY THE LIGHT IT GIVES, MAKE SOMETHING WONDERFUL OF YOUR LIFE

Each person gets all of it—a miracle. Among all our other miracles, there is one particular fact that radio and television bring to the fore, which, for me, opens up whole new fields of speculation. I refer to the fact that hundreds of millions of people (and, of course, billions, if they could be reached) can listen to, or see, *one* broadcast—yet each of them gets all of it, not just a millionth or billionth part, a fractional share! We accept this miracle so casually that we do not even think of it as anything extraordinary. But study it a moment. Give it your conscious attention.

Let me repeat: millions of people hear *one* broadcast, yet each of them gets it in its entirety. Does this not mean, also, that *truth* can be completely present and active in its entirety for each person who conceives it? Does it not mean that God, whatever we conceive Him to be, is completely present and available to each of us? Does it not mean that all *principles* are completely present and available to each of us—entirely so?

Why then is our personal benefit so fragmentary, so seemingly erratic, so occasional? Is it not because our concept is so poor, so limited, fragmentary, and occasional? Why do we live in this world of magnificent powers and know so little about them? Is it because we do not dare to think magnificently—because when largeness presents itself to our minds, we are fearful

224

of it, and shy away, lest the gods become jealous and strike us down? How sad! How tragic!

We'd continue to try to solve our problems in a writhing mass of sense and limitation, when an inner voice is trying to tell us that all we need to lay hold of power is largeness through concept. But we may not bend that power to low uses, for then it turns in upon us and destroys us. We must get very quiet within and obey the "still, small voice" that continually cries of worth and power according to higher laws, the laws of life, being, which are always creating, always becoming, but which bog down when misused. They may not be used, with impunity, AGAINST anyone. They must be used *for* something or somebody.

Movement, Energy, Create and Attract Wealth

The riches of the world are here for man to employ and enjoy. Nature's principles of multiplication almost stagger the human mind. The principle of energy in movement is nowhere better illustrated than in money itself.

Wealth is created by "moving money." Stagnant, piled in a pocket, a drawer, a safe, it remains limited to the amount printed on its face and does not expand in value or service.

Divided among all people, the printed money would give each person only a few dollars. But put that money in circulation and it creates wealth by serving at its face value many times a day.

For instance, start the day with a dollar. Pay it to a taxi driver. The driver pays it to a shoe mender; the shoe mender goes to a movie theatre, and buys popcorn. The popcorn vendor goes to a drugstore and buys a book, a sandwich and a drink. The drugstore pays it to a part-time clerk, who buys two pairs of socks. The merchant buys a ticket to a church social, the church pays its minister, the minister buys gasoline to make calls. The gas-station man buys a chicken from a farmer, the farmer pays his newsboy, the newsboy buys candy and a balloon, the vender buys some ribbon for his baby, etc.

The dollar may change hands fifty to a hundred times a day in an active town. The one dollar is now on record as, say, $100;

for each man must have listed it as income. Thus, moving money is wealth. The faster it moves, the more riches it invokes.

Movement, as we have seen, creates energy. Moving energy becomes a wealth of it! A stagnant man becomes a weak man, just as a stagnant dollar is worth only its face value. In a community where business is stopped, that value may become much, much less.

Start a series of movements. It may be that at this moment, you do not know where to begin to gather energy. The thing to do is to begin with some physical exercises. Get your blood to coursing through your veins. Prepare yourself physically and mentally for a fine life, and do not be thrown off your course by anything or anybody! Move a little, or a great deal, whichever way you must do it. But move *out* negativity and move *in* your clear-cut, fine patterns. Remember all life is movement.

Make a plan for your new life of energy. A plan is a kind of prayer, a vital affirmation. It creates a channel by which your desires may reach you. It also flexes your mental and spiritual muscles. You must have daring. It takes courage to break with the claims of weakness. Write down a plan for yourself. Put into words the way you will spend your energy—and what you expect to get for it.

Build your body wisely and well. Keep it taut and responsive. Give it wonderfully helpful foods and drink. Inform yourself and continually expand your expectation of energy. Breathe deeply of the air, the very atmosphere of well-being.

Treat your mind as though it were a treasure chest. Give no room in it to any soiling or unworthy thing. Gather into it strong, fine inventions and beauties that are rare and fine. Exercise it with reaching concepts. Stretch it to hold the unbelievable promises and wonders of your world and yourself.

Beguile yourself with the melodies of friendship and love. Listen for the tender little things at times. They have much to teach you. When loneliness walks with you, take the stars for companions and let yourself be drawn into the encircling whole of God's great heart, wherein the power to overcome really lives. Thus, your soul will be refreshed and fed and you will step into the world again as a giant.

Start to rise very early. Get up around dawn, and drink in the quiet and the beauty of that time of day. Breathe deeply and invite into your body and mind the riches, beauty and energy of the force behind this new day. Even in fog or rain, there is a newness in the early morning that is potent. Be grateful for it. Dedicate it to fine, strong, "rich" acts and feelings. (You have not time or energy for anything else.) Rest a few minutes later, if you wish.

Meditate on the presence of good ideas, high goals, logical solutions. Bless your enemies, your competitors—for *your* sake, not theirs particularly. This attitude begets an uninhibited flow of energy to and through you.

In the early morning, the very freshness of the day shows up all shoddiness for exactly what it is. Let it alone, and turn *to* all that is worthwhile.

Drink in the pristine worth of the unbelievable power behind this day. Remember, this day is yours. No president, king, or captain can have more. A new day! Bring into it no scar or discord or hurt or weariness from yesterday. Smile on the orderly universe in which everything is in its rightful place—for this is the pattern you desire to bring forth into your own day, and life. Breathe in energy, fresh strength.

You are strong with the indescribable energy of the parent *mind* from which you spring. You are one with this magnificent world, and its forces flow through you. You are vibrant with its magnetisms. You carry a charge of forces of which electricity is only one. You carry forces that we have not as yet discovered! You have areas of potential awareness and extension that are not even known now!

You believe in your inheritance of strength. Oddly enough, though your belief does not change the fact of your inheritance, it does govern your acceptance and use of it.

"It is the Father's good pleasure to give you the kingdom." What does this mean to you? It seems almost too much to assimilate at once. But just try acting as though it were true!

Step out into the world with this feeling of identification with it and calmly accept yourself as a holder of vast energies, so many that you have an overflow for every need you meet, every request. Time, as we have said, seems to stretch out generously when we have great strength with which to use it. When you are rich, you have more of everything than you need for yourself. Live richly and riches follow.

Live from now on in the mature area of abundancies. Turn *from* the law of diminishing returns—*to* the law of accruing force. It is childish, immature, ignorant, blind and animalistic to live and think in terms of punishing limits. Accept them now, if you *must*—but send your mind ahead of your steps into the blessed freedom of the strength, beauty and riches of the world in which you live and move and have your being.

Your life will begin to change. Your body will begin to change. You shall "see" God in your flesh. For *life* and *energy* are *mind*. All change, all creation, begin with concept. Your concept is your pattern for your tomorrows.

How do you see yourself?

INDEX

Index

ABOUT THE AUTHOR

Margery Wilson, well-known counselor on joyous living, well-adjusted personality, and what-is-correct, has been successful in every field she has touched: writing, acting, producing, teaching, lecturing, and the management of business affairs.

Social, home and career obligations, as well as years of study and experience with others have taught her the shortcuts to accomplishment, energy-saving, and emotion and youth-preserving ideas, which she so generously gives to others. *Charm* was Margery Wilson's first book, and since its publication in 1930, she has authored several other publications. She now lives near Los Angeles, but travels extensively on lecture tours.